The American Social Experience Series
GENERAL EDITOR: JAMES KIRBY MARTIN

EDITORS: PAULA S. FASS, STEVEN H.
MINTZ, JAMES W. REED, PETER N.
STEARNS, & ALLAN M. WINKLER

CHILDBEARING IN AMERICAN SOCIETY: 1650–1850

CATHERINE M. SCHOLTEN

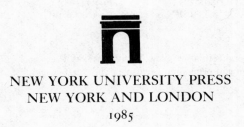

NEW YORK UNIVERSITY PRESS
NEW YORK AND LONDON
1985

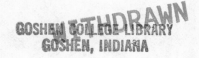

Library of Congress Cataloging in Publication Data

Scholten, Catherine M., 1949–1981.
Childbearing in American society, 1650–1850.

(The American social experience series ; 2)
Bibliography: p.
Includes index.
1. Motherhood—United States—History.   2. Mother
and child—United States—History.   3. Child rearing—
United States—History.   I. Title.   II. Series.
HQ759.S2755   1985   306.8'743'0973   85-322
ISBN 0-8147-7848-8 (alk. paper)

Book design by Ken Venezio

Contents

Preface

This book is an unfinished work that, if completed, would have been a wide-ranging history of childbirth and childrearing in America from the seventeenth century to the 1930s. In its present form, it covers the years up to the 1850s—only about two-thirds of the story Catherine Scholten had hoped to complete but a part that holds great significance for the history of women and the family. During this period, particularly the years from about 1750 to 1830, the experience of giving birth and the task of raising children changed dramatically.

Childbirth, once a frequent event in women's lives, managed by midwives with the help of female relatives and friends, became a much more isolated experience as women had fewer children and male physicians increasingly took over the management of birth. As women had fewer children, the work of raising them assumed much greater importance, and motherhood took on the dimensions of a sacred calling. This book traces the development of these critical changes in the physical practices of childbirth and in methods of raising children, linking both to changes in the status of women in American society.

Catherine Scholten began this book as a Ph.D. dissertation at the University of California at Berkeley. In January 1981, soon after she had finished the third and fourth chapters, she was struck by a car while walking near her home in Berkeley. She suffered massive injuries and died ten days later without having regained consciousness.

Catherine was a native of San Francisco and earned both her B.A. and M.A. degrees in history from Berkeley. In 1971 she received the history department's annual award as its most outstanding undergraduate. Her scholarly interests were broad, encompassing social, urban, medical, and women's history—and she drew on her knowledge of all these fields in writing this book. An earlier version of Chapter 2, published in the *William and Mary Quarterly* under the title "On the Importance of the Obstetrick Art: Changing Customs of Childbirth in America, 1760 to 1825," won that journal's award for the best article published in its 1977 volume. Catherine was also involved in the growth of the new field of oral history; at the time of her death she was an editor for the Regional Oral History Project at the Bancroft Library on the Berkeley campus.

Her family and friends believe that her work, while only a portion of what she had hoped to accomplish, is complete enough in itself to justify publication as a short monograph. What appears in the following pages is essentially Catherine's, with my rather minor rewriting and editing. The conclusion is compiled from the fragments of later chapters that she had written, with some additions to fill out the story. Only the introduction is solely my work. In addition, the notes have been revised to take account of work published since Catherine's death.

Had Catherine lived to publish this book herself, I know she would have thanked, among many others, her mentor at Berkeley, Gunther Barth, her friend Mary Anne Bushman, and the members of her family. I would like to add my own thanks to them for their help and encouragement in preparing Catherine's work for publication. I am especially grateful to her sister, Pauline Scholten, for her help in editing the manuscript and for moral support in what has, at times, been a painful task.

LYNNE WITHEY

San Francisco
May 1984

Introduction

When Abigail Adams gave birth to her first child in 1765, she wrote gleefully to her friends about her new role as a mother. Once over her initial excitement about her new baby, however, she faced the prospect of motherhood with some apprehension, for she firmly believed that mothers were responsible for molding their children into well-educated, virtuous citizens. She, and other women, might expect help from their husbands, schools, and churches, but ultimately the responsibility for their children's moral, intellectual, and psychological development was theirs alone.

Abigail looked to her friend Mercy Otis Warren—sixteen years her senior—for advice, asking her to assist "a young and almost inexperienced Mother in this Arduous Buisness, that the tender twigs allotted to my care, may be so cultivated as to do honour to their parents and prove blessing[s] to the riseing generation." Mercy, however, was appalled at the thought of giving advice on so difficult a task; she herself was "yet looking abroad for Every foreign aid to Enable her to the discharge of a duty that is of the utmost importance to society," she told Abigail.[1]

Their exchange was only one of many that Abigail had with her sisters and friends. Acutely aware of the responsibilities of motherhood, they exchanged books of advice about childrearing and shared with each other their ideas and fears about being mothers. Their concern was a product both of their views about women's domestic responsibilities and also of their ideas about human development. Children, they believed, were innocent, malleable creatures, whose minds and personalities would be molded according to the training and care they received in their early years. The childrearing literature that Abigail read often likened children to plants—plants that had to be "raised and cultivated" carefully. As the "plants" spread, according to one author, they would diffuse "virtue and happiness through the human race."[2]

Such ideas were relatively new in Abigail's time. Older views of children portrayed them as inherently sinful and emphasized the importance of breaking a child's will, preferably by age two, in order to instill habits of obedience. Such ideas were particularly widespread in early New England, where the Calvinist belief in original sin gave strong support to such notions about childrearing. By the time Abigail Adams was raising her children, these older ideas were giving way to the newer belief in childish innocence, although—as in any time—conflicting theories about children and how to raise them existed side by side.

As Catherine Scholten demonstrates in her work, new ideas about childrearing that gained credence in the late eighteenth century had a profound influence on women's lives. Women, of course, had always had the primary responsibility for the care of young children; and women, by implication, bore the responsibility for their well-being and future development. The new emphasis on personal growth and development in raising children elevated women's traditional role as mothers to greater importance, but it also placed a special burden on them, for these theories left little to heredity or chance, placing the responsibility for a child's ultimate character squarely on its mother. A woman might claim much of the credit for her child's achievements, but she also shared in the blame for its failure. Both Abigail Adams and Mercy Warren learned this bitter lesson. When one of Mercy's sons had a nervous breakdown, she was so distraught that she could not bring herself to talk about it, even to Abigail. And Abigail herself, whose firstborn son became president of the United States, fought with her feelings of guilt when her second son died an alcoholic at the age of thirty-one.

Abigail Adams and her friends were unusual in that they embraced the role of motherhood in a highly self-conscious way some time before most other women did. The exaltation of motherhood, so widespread in modern times, first appeared in the years after the Revolution and grew in the early decades of the nineteenth century—hand in hand with changes in the customs and practices of childbirth and in society's perceptions of women in general. This book tells the story of these changes and their relation to each other; as Scholten explains, they did not affect all women in all parts of America at the same time. Eastern, urban, well-educated women like Abigail Adams adopted new ideas and practices long before many other women did—and therefore her life and thoughts offer some clues about the direction that other women would eventually follow.

Although she was one of the first women to adopt some of these new ideas and practices, Abigail Adams in many ways remained rooted in the customs and attitudes of the past. Consequently, her experiences demonstrate something of the complexity of the transition from traditional to modern notions about birth and motherhood.

Abigail bore all her children at home, depending on the assistance of her sisters and close friends during her lying-in, just as women always had; but she also employed a physician, a practice that was new in the late eighteenth century. She believed that women should not have too many children, in keeping with her conviction of the importance of each individual child, and yet she believed in large families— or what would be considered large families by modern standards. On the one hand, Abigail clearly practiced some form of birth control (aided by her husband's long absences during the Revolution); but, after five children, she and John still wanted a sixth, and Abigail conceived a child in 1776, despite the problems of her earlier pregnancies, the uncertainties of war, and the probability that John would be away from home when the child was born. Years later, when she visited France, Abigail was appalled to find that women there commonly limited their families to two or three children. Although she believed that women ought not to bear more children than they could reasonably hope to care for, she also believed that it was women's mission in life to raise children. Eight or nine children might be more than a mother could hope to handle, but surely a mother who had only two or three was shirking her duty.

In other, more subtle ways, Abigail also displayed her links with the past. As deeply attached as she was to her children, and as important as she thought a mother's influence was, she nevertheless sent her children away from her—sometimes for extended periods—when she thought that doing so was best for their welfare. It was a time-honored New England custom to send children to stay with friends or relatives for long stretches; one historian of the colonial family attributes it to the Puritans' desire not to spoil their children.[3] By Abigail's time this practice was less common, but vestiges of it survived; in her case, it was not so much a concern about spoiling her children but her desire to see them become well-educated, well-rounded, independent adults that encouraged her to send them away from home occasionally. As a child she herself had spent long, happy weeks with her grandmother and with her aunt and uncle, and it seemed perfectly natural that her own children should have the same kind of experience.

When the local schools shut down during the Revolution, Abigail sent her sons to live with her sister Elizabeth in another part of the state so that her brother-in-law could prepare them for college. When John went to Europe on a diplomatic assignment during the Revolutionary War, she agreed to his suggestion that he take John Quincy with him. It cost her dearly to part with her son, but she believed that the opportunity for him to see some of the world was too important for a mother's feelings to stand in the way. When John returned to Europe on a second mission, she agreed that both John Quincy and her second son, Charles, should go along. With her sons gone, she felt the need of her daughter's companionship even more keenly; and yet she sent her away to school in Boston for a period of time and to Mercy Warren's home for extended visits, convinced that Mercy would be a valuable influence.

Abigail not only sent her own children away when she thought it would be good for them; she also took in other children occasionally. When her sister Elizabeth had problems with her daughter Betsey, Elizabeth sent her to Abigail, believing that a "new mother" for a while would have a positive effect on her daughter. When Abigail's brother was troubled with severe financial problems, she took in his two-year-old daughter—and ended up raising the child as her own. And when her son Charles died, she did the same for his daughter. To Abigail, there was nothing inconsistent about her belief in the importance of a mother's care and her practice of sending children to stay with friends or relatives. If a mother succeeded in instilling good habits and values in her children at an early age, separation from her later would only serve to broaden their minds and strengthen their independence.

Women of later generations, however, would not necessarily agree. Abigail herself ran into conflict with her daughter-in-law, John Quincy's wife Louisa, on this issue. When John Quincy was elected to the Senate and spent about half the year in Washington and the other half at home in Massachusetts, both he and Abigail thought it best that his sons remain in New England, live with Abigail's sister Mary, and attend a nearby school. The atmosphere in Washington was not conducive to raising children, Abigail believed, and the traveling back and forth would be hard on them. It would be much better for the children to stay with their aunt and uncle—and close by their grandparents—who would give them the best care and see that their education was not interrupted. Louisa, however, disagreed completely; she felt that she had been railroaded into giving up her children by her husband and mother-in-law. She wanted her children with her constantly; she alone would bear the responsibility for them. It was testimony to the strength of her convictions that she successfully fought her highly opinionated, strong-willed mother-in-law and regained control of her children.

These changing attitudes about childbearing and childrearing—attitudes that placed primary emphasis on women's importance as mothers—were intimately linked with a general improvement in women's status in society: this is one of the major themes of Scholten's book. It is a controversial point; historians (and others) have long argued that colonial women enjoyed more independence than did their sisters of later generations and that the nineteenth-century emphasis on motherhood and domesticity served only to diminish women's status and importance in society.

Recently, this belief has come under attack from historians who believe that increasing opportunities for education and the easing of legal restrictions on women in the first half of the nineteenth century indicate an improvement, rather than a decline, in women's condition.[4] Scholten extends this reinterpretation, arguing that the new emphasis on women as mothers was in itself an improvement in women's status because it accorded them a greater measure of respect than they had enjoyed before and elevated them to a position of tremendous influence within the family. She further explains that improvements in women's education, legal status, and position within the family all reinforced each other. Better education for women was justified on the ground that it would make them better mothers; the changes in legal restrictions gave them more control over their children. By analyzing the complex set of reasons for women's increasingly important role as mothers, and the consequences of that role, Scholten illuminates much broader changes in women's position in American society in the nineteenth century.

Ironically, while these changes improved women's status compared with what it had been in the colonial period, they also created a new rationale for placing limits on women's independence. The very arguments that were used to accord new status and respect to women carried with them their own set of restrictions. The argument that women needed to be better educated in order to be good mothers opened new educational opportunities for them, but by sidestepping the issue of women's intellectual capacities and creating a purely practical justification for their education, it also placed limits on the extent of that education. Granting women the status of mistress of the household gave them greater influence within the family circle, but made it even easier to justify limiting their influence outside it.

Abigail Adams, even while she supported the social changes that emphasized women's role as mothers, recognized the pitfalls of these changes. A firm believer in eighteenth-century theories of natural rights and a canny political thinker, she understood that moral influence and status within the family by themselves were not enough to bring about real changes in women's lives. She agreed with the notion that women must be better educated in order to educate their children, but she did not use it as the basis for her arguments that women's education should be improved. Rather, she argued that women were men's intellectual equals and that they had a *right* to an education; improving themselves as mothers would be an additional benefit.

Even more significantly, she understood the importance of legal and political equality. "Remember the Laidies," she said in her most famous statement; "Do not put such unlimited power into the hands of the Husbands. Remember all Men would be tyrants if they could." Half-jokingly, she added, "If perticuliar care and attention is not paid to the Laidies we are determined to foment a Rebelion, and will not hold ourselves bound by any Laws in which we have no voice, or Representation."[5] At the time of the Revolution, talk of natural rights and rebellion was part of everyone's vocabulary; and for intelligent, thoughtful women like Abigail Adams, it seemed perfectly logical to link ideas about natural rights and political independence to perceptions of their own work as wives and mothers. Later generations of women would expand these ideas about women, motherhood, and domesticity but would lose sight of the goal of political and social equality. In the process, they helped place limits on the extent of that improvement.

CHAPTER I

"Daughters of Eve": Women as Childbearers: 1650–1750

"A mother with a train of children after her is one of the most admirable and lovely Sights in the visible Creation of God," declared Benjamin Colman as he introduced the text of his sermon "Fruitful Mothers in Israel" to his Boston congregation. In 1715 the Old Testament injunction "Be fruitful and multiply," which Colman proceeded to discuss, was familiar to his listeners, and his interpretation of the text was representative of American thought on the purpose of marriage and on women's ordained part as childbearer.[1]

American women in the seventeenth and early eighteenth centuries were prolific childbearers, much more so than their European contemporaries or American women of more recent times. Their high birthrates were in part the result of the material conditions of colonial American life—especially the widespread availability of land and the scarcity of labor—but it also reflected a set of social and religious attitudes that viewed childbearing as women's divinely ordained mission in life. Such attitudes were rooted in western European beliefs about the nature of women, but they took on a special meaning in Puritan-

dominated New England, where the biblical view of women reinforced deepseated social attitudes. Ministers often talked of childbearing as the legacy of the "curse of Eve," and their pronouncements frequently betray a callous disregard for the well-being of women and
children. At the same time, however, childbearing conferred a certain
status on women. New mothers were pampered for as much as a month,
the center of attention among friends and family; and women with many
children—and, later, grandchildren—enjoyed special respect and admiration.[2]

Women themselves, although they did not share ministers' views
about the curse of Eve and readily admitted their lack of enthusiasm
for pregnancy, nevertheless generally accepted their role as childbearer. Few tried to limit their pregnancies by birth control or abortion. They did, however, control the conditions surrounding childbirth itself: birth was a thoroughly feminine event, managed by a
midwife with the assistance of the lying-in woman's female relatives
and friends. Their customs of childbirth reveal much about the social
values shaping women's lives in colonial America—both the attitudes
about women and their views of themselves.

Travelers to America in the colonial period were impressed with the
large numbers of children they saw. One visitor remarked that even
"Women from other Places who have been long Married and without
Children" became "joyfull Mothers" in America, and colonial brag-
garts proclaimed, "Our Land free, our Men honest, and our Women
fruitful."[3] Benjamin Franklin's more analytical mind discerned, about
1751, that the American population doubled approximately every
twenty years, independent of immigration. Thomas Malthus, who derived his principle of population from observation of the British North
American colonies, calculated the same rate of growth and termed it
"probably without parallel in history."[4]

The estimates of each woman's contribution to population growth
were, until recently, based on impressions. Historian Arthur Calhoun, relying on randomly gathered genealogies, considered that families of ten to twelve children were "very common" and that families
of twenty to twenty-five children were "not rare enough to call forth
expressions of wonder."[5] Subsequent statistical studies of colonial
communities show that Calhoun's estimates were exaggerated, but even

so, the average woman gave birth to about eight children between her twentieth and fortieth years.[6] This was the highest average rate of birth in American history and was, as Franklin and Malthus correctly observed, higher than contemporary European birthrates.[7]

Why did colonial American women have so many more children than their European contemporaries, or American women in more recent times? Franklin and Malthus—and many others since—attributed the high birthrate to distinct American patterns of land and labor distribution, which lowered the age of marriage. Cheap land and a political system favorable to property ownership meant that no part of the society could have any fears about providing amply for a family by farming. American marriages, Franklin thought, took place earlier than European ones because there was no need for most males to endure a prolonged period of servitude before accumulating the means to support a family. And, by increasing the years of a woman's sexual activity, early marriage increased the number of children she bore.[8]

In general, these explanations are persuasive, although in nineteenth-century America there is reason to doubt a direct correlation between free land and high birthrates. Historians who have compared urban and rural fertility have discovered that the decline in the American birthrate began about 1810, before the United States was statistically an urban nation, and urban and rural fertility declined simultaneously.[9] Independent of conditions in the nineteenth century, statistics do bear out the old assumption that colonial women married early, at the age of twenty-one or twenty-two, which was indeed younger than women in contemporary English agriculture communities.[10]

The corollary to the classic argument that American fertility was related to land use is that children were an asset in the labor-scarce colonies. As one pamphleteer observed, children increased so well in America that they would soon supply the lack of servants. Certainly child labor was "a social fact, not a social problem," and six- and seven-year-old children performed chores of household manufacturing and farming in their own families or as apprentices.[11]

Whether colonial American women and their husbands *consciously* bore children for these reasons is doubtful, however. Certainly they understood the value of children as laborers, and parents also hoped that children would support them in their age or infirmity. The New England Puritans who outlined the reciprocal duties of parent and child termed children "comforts in age" and "a Safe-guard and Protection to us as they grow up."[12] Within this context, the high incidence of child death through accident and disease probably also encouraged procreation. Entries such as William Allason's fill journals throughout the colonial period. My wife "brought me a fine Boy," wrote Allason in 1774, "but poor fellow he stayed only 26 days with us, and made an Exchange much for the better."[13] Mortality rates for children under age ten approached 50 percent throughout the colonies during the middle of the eighteenth century. In his essay on population Benjamin Franklin performed the elementary arithmetic: if a marriage produced eight children, four would grow up.[14]

But it is clear that there are no simple correlations between material conditions and population growth. The availability of land, sustenance, and labor, and the incidence of wealth and mortality do not alone explain the frequency of childbearing, especially in the American case.[15] We must consider too the power of abstractions, in particular those social values that encouraged childbearing in the face of maternal exhaustion.

A range of social values potentially affecting fertility suggests itself—political goals, personal hopes for social and economic improvement, limited concern for women and children as individuals, religious conviction that procreation was God's will. The status of women has ultimate significance, however. Without question, the burden of fecundity fell on colonial women. In a situation where there was little political or economic reason to restrain birth, the high rate of birth reflects the limits of social concern for women and is evidence of the pervasive assumption that frequent childbearing was woman's natural lot and her primary social contribution.

In colonial society all moral authorities agreed that procreation was a divine command.[16] Like their European counterparts, the authors of American sermons and manuals on domestic relations invested the command to multiply with layers of meaning. Childbearing did not continue the species in a mere biological sense; it also meant that there would be a legitimate succession of men created in God's image, and of his commonwealth.[17] Children were his blessings, "among the Choice

Favours and Gifts of Providence," and instruments of his design. Ministers stressed the folly of presuming that any birth occurred independently of divine will. Each child was a servant of Christ, perhaps destined to perform a unique task. "Who knows but that this child may be an eminent instrument to God's glory, a vessel of use in his generation, and a blessing to the whole family?" ran the rhetorical question. The person who attempted to control childbearing tampered dangerously with the divine plan. Those who carried themselves "graciously" if their house filled with children served the Lord.[18]

Women, theologians argued, especially ought to welcome pregnancy as a "merciful visit" of the Lord, a sign of his blessing, and an opportunity to cooperate in their own redemption. In sermons to women, ministers reconciled the two seemingly disparate revelations that childbearing was at once an honor and a curse. It was the "first privilege of the Sex" to carry the "living soul" of the child. Cotton Mather suggested that women derived "more than a little" of their dignity from maternity, for "the Redeemer was *Borne* of a woman"; and Benjamin Colman called pregnancy the "Honour of our first Mother Eve."[19]

Although ministers saluted mothers in their congregations with "Blessed are you among women," they also depicted the pains of childbirth as the appropriate special curse of "the Travailing Daughters of Eve." Women inherited the punishment for Eve's transgression. If the sorrows of childbirth were evidence of sin, the New Testament indicated that they might also be a means of salvation. Ministers followed Paul's word that woman "shall be saved in childbearing if she continued also in faith and charity." They also thought that women's fear of death in childbirth was a mercy, because the "excesses of Piety" that followed "secures for them Eternal Blessedness."[20]

These formal religious explications are the most elegant expression of a mentality that perceived frequent childbearing as woman's ordained lot. Cotton Mather might puzzle through scripture and, with doctrinal precision, tell women that it was "unnatural in you to complain of a state, whereunto the Laws of Nature, established by God, have brought you."[21] Lesser minds bypassed the intricate reasoning and took scripture plainly. Thus, a popular medical manual explained simply that women bring forth children in pain because of God's curse on Eve and reminded readers that the prime purpose of the sacrament of marriage was the production of offspring.[22] Whatever mixture of faith and reason led people to accept scripture literally, the social consequences for women were constant. Their expectations and their behavior were limited. "I do believe women have nothing in the general in view but the breeding contests at home," Virginia gentleman Landon Carter wrote in 1772. "It began with poor Eve and ever since then has been so much of the devil in woman."[23]

Understandably, women viewed the matter in different perspective. Although they accepted frequent childbearing as inevitable, few went so far as to embrace the statement of some ministers that they should welcome childbirth as their divinely ordained mission. On the contrary, some indicated that childbearing sapped them; and well it did, since the average woman spent about six years of her life pregnant, and eight more years nursing infants if they survived. The weariness of Mary Clap, wife of Thomas Clap, president of Yale College, surfaces even through the ritual phrases of her elegy. "She always went thro the Difficulties of Childbearing with a Remarkable Steadiness Faith Patience and Decency, She Had Calm and Humble Resignation to the Divine will," her husband remembered. "Indeed She would Sometimes Say to me that Bearing tending and Burying Children was Hard work, and that She Had Done a great Deal of it for one of Her Age (She Had 6 Children whereof she buried 4 and Dyed in ye 24 year of Her age.)" President Clap missed the point after his wife's death, as he had during her life, for he continued, "Yet [she] would Say it was the work She was made for, and what god in his providence Had Called Her to."[24] Elizabeth Drinker, a Philadelphia Quaker, probably echoed the sentiments of most women when she reflected, "I have often thought that women who live to get over the time of Child-bareing, if other things are favourable to them, experience more comfort and satisfaction than at any other period of their lives."[25]

Undoubtedly many colonial women shared Drinker's sentiments, but few of her contemporaries attempted to limit the frequency of pregnancy. Ministers complained that it was a "folly tho common" among those with many children "to wish and resolve to have no more, and to be cast down with grief and anxious care if they find themselves with child again."[26] But in fact the high rates of birth and the few

public accounts of abortion, infanticide, and contraceptive practice indicate that control of birth was not significant in colonial America. Only
in the late eighteenth century do American population statistics ex-
hibit the characteristics of deliberate family limitation.[27]

This lack of any widespread practice of family limitation was not
the result of lack of knowledge about methods of birth control. In England and France, women were voluntarily limiting birth by the beginning of the eighteenth century, and infanticide was recognized as a
serious problem.[28] European physicians, theologians, and social critics
recorded popular methods of birth control, which were often circulated as folk wisdom.[29] Americans knew the European lore of contra-
ceptives and abortifacients, and scattered evidence suggests that women
occasionally attempted to use them. At trials for attempted abortion
several women admitted to drinking "potions of Physic" and concoc-
tions of the herb savin, a well-known supposed abortifacient.[30]

Landon Carter's daughter-in-law attempted to induce abortion by
trauma. Carter grumbled after one of her miscarriages that she was "a
distressed but really undeserved woman" because the abortion "is her
own fault, a woman that hardly moves when not with child, always
is jolting in a chariot when with child. This is the 3rd destroyed in
this way."[31] There are occasional accounts of coitus interruptus, a more
effective technique than the various potions recommended by folklore.
More common was the practice of breast-feeding children for a year
or longer with the hope of delaying pregnancy. There is medical evidence that suckling inhibits ovulation, and colonial women, observing
the infertility of some nursing mothers, consciously protracted breast-
feeding. Mrs. Carter, in addition to attempting abortion, nursed her
baby "because she should not breed too fast," and the women of the
Drinker family in Philadelphia considered the death of a newborn child
particularly sad because it meant that the mother would "pass through
childbirth a year the sooner."[32] Prolonged lactation was an uncompli-
cated, acceptable means for women to control birth.

However, Americans did not seriously concern themselves with
controlling birth until the nineteenth century. Prolific mothers ful-
filled the laws of God and nature. Benjamin Colman's warning, "Do
not despise the Neighbor who is not blessed" with children, conveys
the stigma of barrenness in the seventeenth and eighteenth centuries.

Even more alien to our twentieth-century sensibility are the words Colman addressed to those with one or two children, "not to envy those with more."[33]

The frank attitude that childbirth was a natural condition for women, and the public character of birth, were evidenced in its prelude, pregnancy. Colonials did not treat pregnancy as an abnormal or shameful condition. Though they recognized it as a special condition, physiologically halfway between sickness and health, and emotionally as a source of anxiety, nothing approaching a rigorous medical course of prenatal care existed in the seventeenth and eighteenth centuries. Medical concern with pregnancy was slight, and social treatment of it matter of fact.

The very language of pregnancy was straightforward. "My wife was indisposed with breeding and very cross," William Byrd wrote in 1712, directly describing his wife's condition. Until the nineteenth century pregnant women were commonly described as "breeding" or "teeming," colloquially as well as in medical literature. The use of the word "breeding" to describe the hatching or birth of animals parallels its application to humans; that it lingered longest in speech in the American South, where fertile or pregnant black slaves were called "breeding women," is an indication of the animalistic implications of the word.[34]

There were no maternity clothes to distinguish pregnancy. Women wore the same garments throughout their life, altering skirt and bodice to their changing size by shifting tapes, laces, and buttons. From about 1600 to 1800 women more often wore a two-piece dress. The skirt, with a drawstring waist or an open front and a separate bodice, laced or overlapped at the front, could be expanded easily to fit a large abdomen. If they followed conventional wisdom or the dictates of a midwife, women removed the corset worn underneath, rather than merely loosening its lacing.[35]

The fashionable robes and sacques also accommodated pregnant waistlines. English women of the seventeenth century were fond of sleeveless robes, which they wore over a loose, highwaisted underdress; and in the eighteenth century stylish women wore the French sacque, a gown that hung uninterruptedly from shoulders to feet, resembling a tent. This dress, especially comfortable during pregnancy, was considered proper for travel and formal occasions.[36]

Indeed, the popularity of the sacque, a garment that would later be considered a robe suitable only for the bedroom, is another indication of the openness of private life. It was acceptable for a pregnant woman to loosen the strings of her bodice, thereby exposing her chemise to the world, or to wear a dressing gown outside the house, because there was at this time no clear distinction between lingerie and streetwear. Undergarments were part of the costume worn under the outer garment, not necessarily clothes to be hidden, and a nightgown was a garment worn during the evening, not merely in bed. This flexible use of garments meant that pregnant women could be comfortable in loose clothes in public.[37]

Women, the bulk of their pregnancy unconcealed, continued their normal activities until shortly before delivery unless a significant crisis, such as a severe fall or vaginal bleeding, compelled bed rest. They undertook journeys by horseback when advanced in pregnancy. They paid social calls and even assisted at the childbirth of friends when their own delivery was but a few weeks away. Pregnancy did not prevent housekeepers from overseeing the slaughter and salting down of pigs in the February weather of New England; nor did it keep weavers from their looms until two to three weeks before their lying-in.[38]

This behavior did not contradict medical wisdom. Midwives and doctors simply advised women not to exercise violently, not to ride in "a Coach that Shakes" or lift any great weights in the first or last months of pregnancy, and to rest when fatigued. These measures, if followed, would not disrupt the lives of most women.[39] Medical literature did not outline a strict regimen of prenatal care but recommended moderate exercise and plain diet and suggested a few palliatives for common complaints of pregnancy. The drama of birth and the lying-in afterward commanded more attention than did the quiet process of pregnancy. Women were more likely to live bound by common fancies and knowledge about pregnancy than by the counsel of physicians. This modest concern with pregnancy indicates the limits of medical interest, knowledge, and practice.

Professional medical authority did not weigh strongly in the colonies. The colonial environment exaggerated what was typical in rural England: untrained men and women practiced medicine as emergencies occurred. A few educated immigrant physicians worked in cities;

some men traveled to Europe to study and others apprenticed themselves to practicing physicians, but overall, the untrained doctored part-
time. As learned men, ministers were often called to prescribe for their
parishioners. However, the first, and often the last, resort were the
home remedies that everyone used liberally. The midwife, a woman
usually qualified by experience rather than by education, treated
women's problems. These conditions of practice meant that medical
care generally was sought only in the crisis of birth. Plainly it had not
occurred to anyone, and no one was encouraging, regular medical
monitoring of pregnancy out of professional interest.[40] In any case,
the learned offered relatively little enlightenment on pregnancy.

The first printed study of midwifery in English, *The Byrth of Man-
kynde*, a translation of the *Rosengarten* written by a Frankfurt physician, appeared in 1540. It was superseded in the following century by
a few handbooks on midwifery that were either translations of Continental works or the productions of self-styled doctors, midwives, and
a few physicians. These books contained the same mixture of occult
notions and Greek pathology that marked early modern medicine in
general.[41]

About the most that could actually be claimed for medical practice
up to about 1750 was that it provided psychological support for the
sick, amelioration of minor ills, treatment of structural injuries, and
occasional quarantine to prevent the spread of contagious disease. The
few truly scientific contributions to medicine of the seventeenth century, such as William Harvey's studies of circulation, which used experimental and quantitative methods to reveal the function of the body,
interested most physicians only tangentially and did not significantly
affect the practice of medicine in Europe or America. Occult notions,
astrology, and classical humoral theory persisted as explanations for
disease. Most practitioners continued to assume that good health depended upon a balance of body fluids (humors), blood, bile, and phlegm,
and they sought to cure disease by depleting excess impure fluids by
inducing bleeding, purging, or vomiting.[42]

When doctors and midwives speculated on fetal development, they
based their guesses on humoral theory, as well as on common lore
and their own observations. They defined pregnancy as an unstable
state in which the humors balanced precariously between sickness and

health, and they attributed complaints of pregnancy, such as nausea and vomiting, to an excess of humors. Some problems of pregnancy could be explained through the principle of association, a key aspect of humorial theory. Violent physical activity, or spasms of the gut, shook loose the embryo and caused abortion. It seemed obvious that a lean diet would starve the fetus.[43]

The fundamental mysteriousness of the physiology of pregnancy is evidenced in the mixtures of explanations presented in the guides of Nicholas Culpeper. Culpeper, who wrote one of the most widely used manuals, described the chapter on the formation of the child in the womb in his *Directory for Midwives* as "the difficultest piece of work in the whol Book, nay in the whol study of Anatomy." Culpeper offered as an excuse the rarity of pregnant corpses for dissection. He had seen only one and claimed that his authorities, Galen and Vesalius, "never saw a woman anatomized." From his observations and reading, Culpeper knew the gross structure of the pelvic organs and the stages of labor, but his embryology was fanciful. He thought that the child was nourished in the womb by menstrual blood and that its growth was governed by the planets, speculations common not only to the authors of popular medical works but also to educated physicians.[44]

On the basis of their admittedly vague understanding of pregnancy, physicians and midwives offered guesses disguised as advice. They focused on preventing abortion by avoiding upsetting extremes in exercise and diet. Hence they counseled against violent exercise and recommended abstention from sexual intercourse during the first months of pregnancy. They proposed a simple diet of plainly cooked meats, wheat bread, green vegetables, and ripe fruits. Highly seasoned foods, with garlic, onions, mustard, and pepper, were to be avoided because they excited the stomach, always weak in pregnancy, and might thereby cause abortion. Apples and dried fruits were recommended to "keep the belly loose," as straining at stool would also lead to abortion. Though the underlying reasoning was faulty, these dietary recommendations reduced two common discomforts of pregnancy, heartburn and constipation, and were reasonably sound by modern standards of nutrition.[45]

Some specific remedies, still honored for complaints of pregnancy, were recorded in the literature, such as the suggestion that women with varicose veins in their legs rest with their feet elevated and that those suffering with hemorrhoids apply warm polutices to the afflicted area. However, the more abstract problems of preventing miscarriage or causing an easy birth received more magic treatment. There were herbs and spices that supposedly would "strengthen the womb," among them sage ale, drunk in the morning, and nutmeg and cloves, applied to the navel. Wearing minerals and gems, particularly in a lodestone or a piece of coral, would hold a child in the womb. Conversely, removal of these from the body would hurry labor.[46] Other suggestions likely originated in the associative faculties of the human imagination. Women who would ease their labor were advised to drink "Sallet oyl" and to anoint the birth place with oil of lilies or capon's grease throughout pregnancy.[4]

How carefully women heeded these prescriptions is impossible to know. Certainly it was common knowledge that a sensible pregnant woman avoided extremes of diet and motion. Hence, Landon Carter thought that his pregnant daughter-in-law "intended to forward abortion" by eating heartily of inappropriate foods and understood, correctly, that she hoped to abort herself by bouncing along Virginia roads in her carriage. Other prohibitions were generally known. Careful or clever women felt that they could rightfully demand cessation of sexual intercourse during pregnancy, though others, as we know from divorce petitions, merely cautioned husbands to "use them gently" when they were with child.[48] The precautions that women did take were not part of a supervised schedule of pregnancy care, as women did not consult midwives unless they had a specific problem. Some warned midwives a few weeks before their expected date of confinement, and those in the country, with means, might board the midwife for the days near their anticipated delivery; but generally the midwife was called only at the time of labor.[49]

The vagueness of prenatal care in the medical literature and the absence of a consistent routine of care imply that colonial Americans considered pregnancy an ordinary event. However, in recognizing that pregnancy was ordinary, we should be careful not to diminish the anxieties that it created. Inordinate concern with "longings of pregnancy" and "marking the child," and descriptions of pregnant women as unstable, hysterical, and fearful tell us that childbearing disturbed many women.

Pregnant women worried that they might harm their unborn child, for it was a common conviction that sudden frights, strong passions, or ungratified longings for peculiar things would disfigure the child. The theory that a mother can impress her child is an ancient explanation for hereditary deformities and character traits, which persists today on what the educated term the "folk" level. Through the nineteenth century, authority verified what everyone supposed—that trauma marked the child. If a pregnant woman looked upon "terrible things," or was startled by a loud noise, the child would be marked. Undoubtedly, a hare jumping quickly in front of a woman caused harelip.[50] Cotton Mather speculated that the fright of "an horrible Spectre" that his wife saw on their porch a few weeks before her delivery in 1693 caused their child to be born malformed, and women of the neighborhood confirmed that this was the reason.[51]

A woman could do little but worry about he child if she did experience a shock, but it was possible, some thought, to control the equally pernicious longings and passions of pregnancy. The "passions and surfeits" of the mother made strange impressions on the infant, even affecting its soul. Lascivious feelings might cause depravity in the child. It therefore became women to remain "calm and sober," for infants would be "naturally and powerfully affected" by their temperance.[52] Longings, if ungratified, caused abortion or printed the child's body with marks resembling the figure and color of what the mother longed for, an assumption sound enough to be grounds for suit for damages in a seventeenth-century Virginia court. Women usually craved special foods, often out-of-season fruits, but occasionally desired to eat dirt, clay, or chalk. Some shrewd women seized on their advantage and longed for new furniture and clothes, which perhaps led the thoughtful to conclude that women who lived idly or ate poorly suffered longings most frequently. The usual advice was immediate indulgence of the thing longed for if it was not unwholesome. Thus, one manual proposed that beans boiled with sugar be substituted for clay or coal and suggested that if a woman longed for something that she could not obtain, "let her presently drink a large Draught of pure cold water."[53]

The advice to remain calm and sober, and to restrain excessive eating and drinking for the good of the child, probably also represented an attempt to tranquilize the mother for her own sake.[54] The lengthy discussions of longings and markings in midwifery manuals suggest that pregnant women were capricious and emotionally unstable. In fact, men took "hysterick fits" as a sign that a woman "might be breeding."[55] The author of one manual, John Oliver, explained that melancholy; hysterical vapors, pains, and illnesses; and "sad apprehensions of the burthen they carry and the hazard they are in," made it "impossible" for pregnant women "to be in so good a humor as at other times."[56]

Yet Oliver's book could have contributed little to the serenity of the women who read it. Like the other tracts written specifically for lying-in women, Oliver's *Present for Teeming American Women* dwelt on the divinely ordained hazards of childbirth and advised a hearty course of meditation on death. Cotton Mather's pamphlet, *Elizabeth in Her Holy Retirement*, which he distributed to Boston midwives to give to the women they cared for, described pregnancy as a virtually lethal condition. "For aught you know," it warned, "your Death has entered into you, you may have conceived that which determines but about Nine Months more at the most, for you to live in the World." Pregnancy was thus intended to inspire piety.[57]

John Oliver similarly reminded expectant mothers that prayer was necessary because their dangers were many. He noted that women preparing for lying-in "get Linnen and other necessaries for the child, a nurse, a midwife, entertainment for the women that are called to the Labour, a warm convenient chamber, and etc." However, "all these may prove miserable comforters," argued Oliver, for "they may perchance need no other linnen shortly but a Winding Sheet, and have no other chamber but a grave, no neighbours but worms."[58] He counseled women to "arm themselves with patience" as well as with prayer, and, in labor, to "abate somewhat those dreadful groans and cries which do so much discourage their friends and relations that are near them."[59]

Surely women did not need to be reminded of the risks of childbirth; they knew of women who received injury or died giving birth. Though the stereotype of the "slaughter of womanhood in incessant childbearing" in colonial times is exaggerated, women died of complications of childbirth often enough to instill a reasonable fear of birth in the survivors.[60] Statistical representation of general maternal mortality rates before the late nineteenth century is conjecture; mortality bills in which the cause of death is unclear are compounded by incomplete census records. One study of seventeenth-century Plymouth tells us that childbirth was not the major cause of death among women, for a bit less than 20 percent of deaths of adult females were related to childbirth. Still, this means that every fifth woman died of causes associated with childbirth, or one birth in thirty resulted in the death of the mother, a high relation of birth to death, and an association magnified in small communities by intimate knowledge of the circumstances.[61]

Women might survive childbirth but suffer poor health as a consequence. The "serious protracted illness" of Mrs. Henry Laurens worsened with each annual confinement and "cast gloom" over her household.[62] The injury Elizabeth Drinker received during the birth of her ninth child rendered her an invalid and made her acutely sensitive to the troubles of her daughter, who acquired a recto-vaginal tear while giving birth. Molly was thereafter incontinent of feces, and her mother wrote that she was, at the age of twenty-five, "not fit to be around with other people," words that suggest the misery of women with similar tears of bladder, rectum, and vagina, traumas of childbirth that were irreparable until the mid-nineteenth century.[63]

Women anticipated childbirth with dread. Anne Bradstreet expressed her anxiety poetically in a verse she wrote to her husband "Before the Birth of One of Her Children": "How soon, my Dear, death may my steps attend. How soon't may be thy lot to lose thy friend."[64] Mary Clap sought to quiet her fears with prayer and, before each of her six lyings-in, asked her husband to pray with her that God would continue their lives together.[65]

Women facing the hazards of childbirth depended on the community of their sex for companionship and medical assistance. Those who had moved away at marriage frequently returned to their parents' homes for delivery, either because they had no neighbors or because they preferred the care of their mothers to that of their in-laws. Other women summoned mothers, sisters, aunts, and cousins on both sides of the family, as well as female friends, when birth was imminent.[66] Above all, they relied on the experience of midwives to guide them through labor.

Women monopolized the practice of midwifery in America, as in

Europe, through the middle of the eighteenth century. As the recognized experts in the conduct of childbirth, they advised the mother-to-be if any troubles arose during pregnancy, supervised the activities of lying-in, and used their skills to assure safe delivery. Until educated male physicians began to practice obstetrics, midwives enjoyed some status in the medical profession, enhanced by their legal responsibilities in the communities they served.

English authorities required midwives to take oaths in order to be licensed but imposed no official test of their skills. Though originating in the sixteenth century in ecclesiastical anxieties that infants in danger of death be baptized, and that no charms or sorcery be used by midwives to hasten labor, by the eighteenth century the oaths contained many provisions on aspects of public health and welfare. The oaths, which midwives signed in parish registers, indicate that, as the appropriate attendants at birth, midwives had responsibilities serious enough to warrant supervision. As well as swearing not to allow any infant to be baptized outside the Church of England, midwives promised to help both rich and poor, to report the true parentage of a child, and to abstain from performing abortions. Oath-breaking midwives could be excommunicated or fined. Occasionally the conventional oath was supplemented by affidavits attesting to a woman's skill.[67]

Some American midwives learned their art in Europe, where midwifery was almost exclusively the professional province of women. Though barber-surgeons and physicians increasingly asserted their interest in midwifery during the seventeenth century, midwives and patients resisted the intruders.[68] Midwives took pride in their calling, saying that the "holy Scripture hath recorded midwives to the Perpetual Honour of the Female Sex."[69] The midwives of London, who for a time attempted to maintain standards of practice through a system of apprenticeship, in petitions to the Crown in the seventeenth century referred to themselves as "midwives by our profession" and reminded their king that they were "well-paid and highly regarded in our parishes for our great skill and mid-night industry."[70] The author of "Instructions of a Midwife to Her Daughter" elaborated on the duties and ethics of the calling. Use only proven medicines, deliver whores in an honest place, she wrote, and be continually learning to "so increase thy Talent, that people may say you are better than ever your mother was." Above all, she advised, a midwife should remain calm in emergencies, for "a person that keeps her Wits together, without suffering them to be scattered by fear, is capable of giving assistance in weighty affairs."[71]

The midwives' levels of skill varied from the London aspirations and accomplishments. Some women acquired a medical education in the same way as many surgeons and physicians, namely by apprenticeship. Some read manuals by more learned midwives and physicians; and, after 1739, when the first British lying-in hospital was founded, a few were taught by the physicians who directed the hospitals.[72] But, more often than not, women undertook midwifery equipped only with folk knowledge and the experience of their own pregnancies. Country midwives, who sometimes could not read, were singled out as the worst violators of any standards that may have prevailed.[73]

Disparity of skills also existed among American midwives. Experienced midwives, some trained in Europe, practiced alongside women who were, one physician observed, "as ignorant of their business as the women they deliver."[74] By the end of the eighteenth century physicians thought that the "greater part" of the midwives in America took up the occupation by accident, "having first been *catched*, as they express it, with a woman in labour."[75] The more diligent sought help from books, probably popular medical manuals such as *Aristotle's Master Piece*.[76]

American midwives conducted their practice free, on the whole, from governmental supervision. Only two colonies appear to have enacted regulatory statutes, and it does not seem that these were rigorously enforced. In the seventeenth century Massachusetts and New York required midwives, together with surgeons and physicians, not to act contrary to the accepted rules of their art. More specifically, in 1716 the common council of New York City prescribed a licensing oath for midwives, which was similar to the oaths of England, though without the provision on baptism. The oath, significantly, included an injunction that midwives not "open any matter Appertaining to your Office in the presence of any Man unless Necessity or Great Urgent Cause do constrain you to do so."[77] This oath, which was regularly reenacted until 1763, suggests the common restriction of midwifery to women, excluding male physicians or barber-surgeons, who, in any case, were few and usually ill-trained. There are records of male mid-wives in New York, Philadelphia, Charleston, and Annapolis after 1740, but only one, a Dr. Spencer of Philadelphia, had London training in midwifery, and it was said of another that he attended very few natural births.[78]

Though their duties were not as well defined by law, American midwives served the community in ways similar to those of their British counterparts. Early colonists, recognizing the value of having with them a woman whose occupation was to attend births, enticed midwives to settle in their communities by giving them salaries or houses and lots rent-free.[79] For, in addition to assisting at childbed, midwives testified in court in cases of bastardy, verified birth dates, and examined female prisoners who pleaded pregnancy to escape punishment.[80] A few notebooks that survive from the late eighteenth century show us that conscientious midwives recorded the birth date, sex, and names of the parents of the children they delivered.[81] Some colonials also observed the English custom of having the midwife attend the baptism and burial of infants. Samuel Sewall reported that Elizabeth Weeden brought his son John to church for christening in 1677, and at the funeral of little Henry in 1685, "Midwife Weeden and Nurse Hill carried the Corps by turns."[82]

The inclusion of the midwife in these ceremonies of birth and death shows that women valued midwives for more than mere skill. Women with gynecologic problems would freely tell a midwife things "that they had rather die than discover to the Doctor."[83] Grateful patients eulogized midwives.[84] The acknowledgment of the services of one Boston midwife, recorded on her tombstone, had inspired comment since 1761. The stone informs the curious that Mrs. Phillips was "born in Westminster in Great Britain, and Commission'd by John Laud, Bishop of London in ye Year 1718 to ye Office of a Midwife," came to "this Country" in 1719, and "by ye Blessing of God has brought into this world above 3000 Children."[85]

We may picture Mrs. Phillips's professional milieu as a small room, lit and warmed by a large fire, and crowded by a gathering of family and friends. In daytime, during the early stages of labor, children might be present; and while labor proceeded, female friends dropped in to offer encouragement and help. Securing refreshments for the visitors was a part of the preparation for childbirth, especially among the well-to-do.[86] Men did not usually remain in the lying-in room. After traveling throughout the neighborhood gathering the midwife and other women, husbands might be summoned in to pray at the bedside, but as delivery approached they waited elsewhere, with the children and with women who were "not able to endure" the tension in the room.[87]

During the final stages of labor, the midwife took full charge, assisted by other women. Ideally, midwives managed labor by letting nature do the work; they caught the child, tied the umbilical cord, and if necessary fetched the afterbirth. Alcoholic spirits were the only painkillers they gave. Midwives sometimes rubbed the vagina of a woman in labor with butter or oils, believing that this would hasten the dilation of the parts. If labor progressed slowly, midwives could prescribe remedies of dubious efficacy, such as drinks of cinnamon water, swallows' nests dissolved in water, or application of a magnet or horseshoe to the genitals to draw the child out. In complicated cases they might turn the child and deliver it feet first, but if this failed the fetus had to be destroyed. In all circumstances the midwife's chief duty was to comfort the woman in labor while they both waited on nature, and this task she could fulfill with social ease.[88]

As a woman, the midwife managed the events in the lying-in room without embarrassment. While friends laid out childbed linens and readied basins and towels, the midwife made sure that the clothes of the laboring woman were loose and her bowels empty. Under her direction the woman in labor was fortified with hard liquor or mulled wine or was fed broth or eggs if she seemed weak. From time to time the midwife freely examined her cervix to gauge the progress of labor and encouraged her to walk about until the pains became too strong.[89] There was no standard posture for giving birth, but apparently few women lay flat in bed. Some squatted on a midwife's stool, a low chair with an open seat. Others knelt on a pallet, sat on another woman's lap, or stood supported by two friends.[90]

Friends were "welcome companions," according to one manual for midwives, because they enabled the women in labor "to bear her pains to more advantage," and "their cheerful conversation supports her spirits and inspires her with confidence."[91] Elizabeth Drinker endeavored to talk her daughter into better spirits by telling her that as she was thirty-

nine "this might possibly the last trial of this sort."[92] Some women
attempted to cheer the mother-to-be by assuring her that her labor was
easy compared with others they had seen, or they provoked laughter
by making bawdy jokes.[93] The tying of the umbilical cord provided
subject for much discussion, as it was "received opinion" that the size
of an infant's genitals would correspond to the length of the cut cord.
Everyone present at a delivery gave her opinion as to where the cut
would leave a male "well provided for the Encounters of Venus" or
what length would make a female's vagina small enough to please her
husband but large enough for easy childbirth.[94]

Despite the conviviality that might at times prevail, for some attendants a delivery could be a wrenching experience. Elizabeth Drinker
relived her own difficult deliveries when her daughters suffered their
labors, and on one such occasion she noted with irony, "This day is
38 years since I was in agonies bringing her into this world of troubles: she told me with tears that this was her birthday."[95] For others,
assisting at the labors of friends was a reminder of their sex. Sarah
Eve, an unmarried twenty-two-year-old, helped at the labor of a friend
in 1772 and carried the tidings of birth to the waiting father. "None
but those that were like anxious could be sensible of a joy like theirs,"
she wrote in her journal that night. "Oh! Eve! Adam's wife I mean—
who could forget her to-day?"[96]

After delivery the mother was covered up snugly and confined to
her bed, ideally for three to four weeks. By medical reasoning, the
ordeal of birth left the mother seriously debilitated, and the period of
bed rest, her lying-in, protected her while she recovered strength.
Stirring as little as possible in bed for at least three days after giving
birth, and remaining in the house for three weeks more, the new mother
was fed a "strengthening" diet of red meat, eggs, wine, and ale. As
she was thought to be highly susceptible to cold, her room was heated,
her bed was piled with blankets, and she was constantly supplied with
hot drinks.[97] American women with families or hired nurses to relieve
them of household duties, and with room to lie in, actually observed
a month of confinement. Restless women, and those who could not
afford weeks of idleness, got up in a week or less, but not without
occasioning censure for threatening their health.[98]

The exaggerated period of rest following childbirth was medically appropriate, by standards of the time, and it allowed women to establish a routine of breast-feeding, though nurses might assume this responsibility along with other tasks of childcare.[99] However, the lying-in served other purposes too. The long seclusion was associated with the biblical rituals of purification, which an unclean woman performed after childbirth. The Mosaic Law clearly tinges the advices of midwife Jane Sharp, who suggests a longer lying-in if the child is a girl, and who cites the "Time of Purification" as the reason why husbands must then abstain from their wives.[100] More important, the lying-in was the occasion when family and community formally acknowledged the new mother's social contribution. The act of giving birth entitled her to a month of special care and ceremony and was, for most women, the only occasion other than their wedding when they were the focus of attention.

The birth of a child and the safe delivery of its mother attracted many visitors to the lying-in chamber. At times as many as eighteen women crowded by a mother's bed, defeating the medical injunctions that she have silence and rest. Often the new mother treated her midwife and friends to a banquet; such were the feasts of "Boil'd Pork, Beef, Fowls, very good Rost Beef, Turkey-Pye, Tarts" that Mrs. Sewall gave her women days after her delivery.[101] Sometimes guests followed an elaborate protocol of visits. In polite Philadelphia society the mother received only near female relatives and intimate friends during the first week of her confinement. In the second week, the rest of the family and acquaintances came, but no men were admitted until the third week of ceremonious visits.[102] Women in other communities put on their best clothes and carried small gifts to the child during "setting up week," the last week before the mother's "first going out."[103]

Women marked in their diaries the first time they went out of the house, when they reemerged into the world, but their childbirth and confinement had been, in our terms, an open event. Their pains of body and mind during birth had been exposed to neighbors and relatives of all degrees and were hardly secret to the husbands and children who shared the house. The openness of birth was consistent with the generally low standards of personal privacy. Little of what we now call intimate life was hidden in the crowded, poorly partitioned houses of colonial Americans. But the technology of domestic architecture and large families—both material bars to privacy—existed in a social context that discouraged anonymity. Relatives and neighbors in the agricultural, preindustrial communities of New England assumed that they had a right to enter houses without knocking, in order to satisfy their curiosity about any noises or to oversee the potentially immoral activities of others.[104] It was fitting that the community should witness birth too.

Birth was public, but the audience was feminine. John Alexander placed the discussion of childbirth in his history of women under the chapter heading "Customs, for the most part observed only by women," a precise label in the Anglo-American world of the 1770s. Birth was truly, as he termed it, a "sexual ceremony of women," because it was managed and witnessed by women.[105] The prolonged convalescence on special childbed linen and the parties and visits that women enjoyed after birth affirmed the importance of their status as childbearers.

Toward the end of the eighteenth century, however, the customs of childbirth began to change. American women—especially middle-class women living in urban areas and the long-settled regions of the Atlantic seaboard—had fewer children, on the average, than the women of their mothers' and grandmothers' generations; this decline in fertility continued and became more pronounced in the nineteenth century. At about the same time, the distinctly feminine character of childbirth changed also. Men trained in medicine began to study and practice midwifery in increasing numbers, and as they moved into this field they pushed women out, arguing that childbirth was a dangerous and delicate process requiring the expert assistance of a physician. At the same time, they denied women access to the formal training in obstetrics, claiming it as their badge of expertise.

Women at first resisted the employment of men at childbirth, partly because of the psychological association of male physicians with difficult births—the only kind where they were called upon during most of the colonial period—and partly because of feminine modesty and the strong tradition of childbirth as a female event. But gradually middle- and upper-class women were persuaded of the value of expert assistance, believing that birth would be safer and perhaps easier under the guidance of a well-trained man. As a consequence of these changes, by the beginning of the nineteenth century childbirth had become a less frequent, more private, and less exclusively feminine event for a substantial proportion of American women.

CHAPTER 2

The Medical Management of Childbirth: 1760–1825

In October 1799, as Sally Downing of Philadelphia labored to give birth to her sixth child, her mother, Elizabeth Drinker, watched her suffer "in great distress." Finally, on the third day of fruitless labor, Sally's physician, William Shippen, Jr., announced that "the child must be brought forward." Elizabeth Drinker later wrote that, happily, Sally delivered naturally, although Dr. Shippen had said that "he thought he should have occasion for instruments" and clapped his hand on his side so that the forceps rattled in his pocket.[1]

Elizabeth Drinker's account of her daughter's delivery is one of the few written descriptions of childbirth by an eighteenth-century woman. It is of special interest to social historians because it records the participation of a man attending at birth in the capacity of a physician. Shippen was a prominent member of the first generation of American doctors trained in obstetrics and, commencing in 1763, the first to maintain a regular practice attending women in childbirth.[2] With Shippen, male physicians began to supplant midwives.

During the half century after 1770, beginning in Boston, Philadelphia, and New York, male physicians assumed the practice of midwifery among well-to-do women. Initially they entered the field as trained practitioners who could help women in difficult labors, but ultimately they presided over normal deliveries as well. By analyzing the changing social customs and medical management of childbirth from 1760 to 1825 we can identify the emergence of new patterns in private and professional life. The presence of male physicians in the lying-in room signaled a general change in attitudes toward childbirth. With changing conditions of urban life, new perceptions of women, and advancements in medical science, birth became increasingly regarded as a medical problem to be managed by physicians. At the same time, because medical training was restricted to men, women lost their position as assistants at childbirth, and an event traditionally managed by a community of women became an experience shared primarily by a woman and her doctor.

William Shippen quietly overcame resistance to the presence of a man in the lying-in room. Caspar Wistar, in his *Eulogium on Dr. Shippen*, published in Philadelphia in 1818, recalled that when Shippen began in 1763, male practitioners were resorted to only in a crisis. "This was altogether the effect of prejudice," Wistar remarked, adding that "by Shippen this prejudice was so done away, that in the course of ten years he became very fully employed."[3]

A few figures testify to the trend. The Philadelphia city directory in 1815 listed twenty-one women as midwives and twenty-three men as practitioners of midwifery. In 1819 it listed only thirteen female midwives, while the number of men had risen to forty-two; by 1824 only six female midwives remained in the directory.[4] "Prejudice" similarly dissolved in Boston, where in 1781 physicians advertised that they expected immediate payment for their services in midwifery; by 1820 midwifery was almost "entirely confined" to physicians.[5] By 1826 Dr. William Potts Dewees, professor of midwifery at the University of Pennsylvania and the outstanding American obstetrician of the early nineteenth century, could preface his textbook on midwifery with an injunction to every American medical student to study the subject because "everyone almost" must practice it. He wrote that "a change of manners within a few years" had "resulted in almost exclusive employment of the male practitioner."[6]

Dewees's statement must be qualified because the "almost exclusive" use of men actually meant almost exclusive use among upper- and middle-class urban women, or what Dr. Walter Channing of Boston described as the "richer and better informed." Female midwives continued throughout the nineteenth century to serve both the mass of women in cities and women in the country who were, as Channing put it, "without the advantage of regular practitioners."[7] During the initial years of their practices, physicians shared obstetrical cases with midwives. On occasion Philadelphia women summoned Shippen together with their midwives, and Dewees reported that when he began to practice in the 1790s he depended on midwives to call him when instruments were needed.[8] It is clear, however, that by the 1820s Dewees and his colleagues had established their own practices independent of midwives.

The change was, in part, a consequence of the fact that after 1750 growing numbers of American men traveled to Europe for medical education. Young men with paternal means, like Shippen, spent three to four years studying medicine, including midwifery, with leading physicians in the hospitals of London and the classrooms of Edinburgh. When they returned to the colonies, they brought back not only a superior set of skills but also British ideas about hospitals, medical schools, and professional standards.[9]

In the latter part of the eighteenth century, advanced medical training became available in North America. At the time of Shippen's return in 1762 there was only one hospital in the colonies, the Pennsylvania Hospital, opened ten years earlier to care for the sick poor. Shippen and his London-educated colleagues saw that the hospital could be used for the clinical training of physicians, as in Europe. Within three years the Philadelphia doctors, led by John Morgan, established formal, systematic instruction at the school of medicine, supplemented by clinical work in the hospital.[10] Morgan maintained that the growth of the colonies "called aloud" for a medical school "to increase the number of those who exercise the profession of medicine and surgery."[11] Dr. Samuel Bard successfully addressed the same argument to the citizens of New York in 1768.[12]

In addition to promoting medical schools, Morgan and Bard defined the proper practitioner of medicine as a man learned in science. Schooled to approach medical problems with a new critical empricism and confident of the natural causes of disease, Morgan and Bard thought of medicine as an experimental science in which theories of disease were substantiated by careful, clinical observation. To master this "intricate science, founded on numberless facts," and unconnected with religion, mystery, and superstition, the ideal physician added anatomy, material medicine, botany, chemistry, and clinical experience to his knowledge of languages and the liberal arts.[13] Thus educated, the physician was highly conscious, not only of his responsibility to preserve "the lives of mankind," but also of the dignity of his profession.[14] This new emphasis on professionalism, affirmed by other American physicians, extended to midwifery.[15]

The trustees of the first American medical schools recognized midwifery as a branch of medical science. From its founding in 1768, King's College in New York devoted one professorship solely to midwifery, and the University of Pennsylvania elected Shippen professor of anatomy, surgery, and midwifery in 1791. By 1807 five reputable American medical schools provided courses in midwifery.[16] In the early years of the nineteenth century some professors of midwifery began to call themselves obstetricians or professors of obstetrics, scientific-sounding titles free of the feminine connotations of the word "midwife."[17] Though not compulsory for all medical students, the new field was considered worthy of detailed study along the paths pioneered by English physicians.

Continental practitioners, notably the French, also began to approach midwifery scientifically in the eighteenth century, but British men led the development of the specialty.[18] British barber-surgeons and physicians long had assisted in labors when extraction of a dead fetus was required, and occasionally compiled texts of advice on midwifery or translated Continental works on the subject.[19] Peter Chamberlen the Elder invented obstetrical forceps—later an important constituent of men's claim to superior technique in midwifery—about 1600, but the men of his family kept secret the design of their instrument through over 100 years of practice in London.[20] The significant changes in the practice of midwifery resulted from the application of the new critical, clinical methods that began to transform medicine as a whole in the eighteenth century. The nature of the new developments, which directly influenced Americans, is exemplified in the work of Dr. William Smellie and his pupils.

Smellie contributed more to the development of obstetrics than any other eighteenth-century physician. His influence was established by his teaching career in London from 1741 to 1758 and by his treatise on midwifery, first published in 1752.[21] Through precise measurement and observation Smellie discovered the mechanics of parturition. He found that the child's head turned throughout delivery, adapting the widest part to the widest diameter of the pelvic canal. Accordingly, he defined maneuvers for manipulating an improperly presented child. He also recognized that obstetrical forceps, generally known for only twenty years when he wrote in 1754, should be used to rectify the position of an infant wedged in the mouth of the cervix, in preference to the "common method" of simply jerking the child out. He perfected the design of the forceps and explained its proper use so that physicians could save both mother and child in difficult deliveries instead of being forced to dismember the infant with hooks.[22]

In his *Treatise* and in his *Anatomical Tables*, Smellie provided a model of his method. He carefully outlined obstetrical technique, substantiating his recommendations with accurate plates and myriad case histories. He continually reminded his readers that they should, as he had, attend to the course of nature and interfere with their hands, instruments, and medicines only as a last resort.[23] Smellie directly impressed his insights on hundreds of students in London, whose own research and teaching enlarged his efforts. Anatomist William Hunter, Shippen's professor, produced in 1774, after thirty years of dissections, a magnificent exposition of the structure of the gravid uterus.[24] Dr. Colin Mackenzie circumvented some of the difficulties Smellie had encountered in finding women to deliver by founding a semiprivate maternity hospital. When Smellie began teaching, man midwives were called for only in desperate cases, which meant that his students hardly ever observed normal labor. The lying-in hospitals that physicians founded in British cities in the last half of the eighteenth century provided medical care for poor women and clinical cases for medical students. At Mackenzie's London hospital it was possible for Shippen to examine seventeen pregnant women in one day and thereby see what he had heard described in lectures.[25]

To Smellie and the men who learned from him, the time seemed ripe to apply science to a field hitherto built on ignorance and supported by prejudice. Smellie commented on the novelty of scientific interest in midwifery. "We ought to be ashamed of ourselves," he admonished the readers of his *Treatise*, "for the little improvement we have made in so many centuries." Only recently have "we established a better method of delivering in laborious and preternatural cases."[26] Smellie's countryman Dr. Charles White reflected in his text on midwifery in 1773 that "the bringing of the art of midwifery to perfection upon scientific and medical principles seems to have been reserved for the present generation."[27]

Some American physicians shared this sense of the new "Importance of the Obstetrick Art." Midwifery was not a "trifling" matter to be left to the uneducated, Thomas Jones of the College of Medicine of Maryland wrote in 1812. Broadly defined as the care of "all the indispositions incident to women from the commencement of pregnancy to the termination of lactation," it ranked among the most important branches of medicine. And, with the cultivation of this branch of science, women could now "reasonably look to men for safety in the perilous conditions" of childbirth.[28]

Jones maintained, as did other physicians, that the conditions of modern urban life produced a special need for scientific aid in childbirth. To a man, they thought that hardy Indian squaws gave birth painlessly but that civilized and refined women endured painful, difficult childbirth. Both rich and poor women in "all populous and wealthy cities" presented troublesome cases to the physician. Jones considered pelvic deformities, abortions, and tedious labors common among wealthy urban women because of their indolent habits and confining fashionable dress and among the poor because of their inadequate diet and long hours of work indoors. Jones cited statistics of maternal mortality and difficult labors from British cities, which he thought revealed how urbanization blighted women's health. Other American doctors agreed, on the basis of their own experience, that there was a greater need for well-informed obstetricians in large cities.[29]

Although it cannot be established that there was an increase in difficult births among urban women, social as well as medical reasons account for the innovations in the practice of midwifery in Boston, Philadelphia, and New York. These were truly populous and wealthy places. The Philadelphia in which Shippen began practice had a population of about 24,000, as large as Edinburgh, where he had studied; Samuel Bard's New York of 1765 had about 18,000 people. When Jones surveyed the American obstetrical scene in 1812, these cities had grown in size and wealth. New York had a population of 96,000, Philadelphia of 54,000; and his Baltimore had 47,000 residents.[30]

These cities supported the medical schools where physicians received medical education and offered the best opportunities to acquire patients and live comfortably. Urban families of some means could afford the $12 to $15 minimum fee that Boston physicians demanded for midwife services in 1806.[31] Obstetrics was found to be a good way to establish a successful general practice. The man who conducted himself well in the lying-in room won the gratitude and confidence of his patient and her family, and they naturally asked him to serve in other medical emergencies. It was midwifery, concluded Dr. Walter Channing of Boston, that ensured doctors "the permanency and security of all their business."[32]

The possibility of summoning a physician, who could perhaps ensure a safer and faster delivery, opened first to urban women. The dramatic rescue of one mother and child given up by a midwife could be enough to convince a neighborhood of women of a physician's value and secure him their practice.[33] Doctors asserted that women increasingly hired physicians because they became convinced "that the well instructed physician is best calculated to avert danger and surmount difficulties."[34] Certainly by 1795 the women of the Drinker family believed that none but a physician should order medicine for a woman in childbed, and they had no doubts that Dr. Shippen or his colleague, Dr. Nicholas Way, were the best help that they could summon.[35]

Although she accepted a male physician as midwife, Elizabeth Drinker still had reservations about the use of instruments to facilitate childbirth and was relieved when Shippen did not have to use forceps on her daughter. Other women feared to call a physician because they assumed that any instruments he used would destroy the child.[36] Once the capabilities of obstetrical forceps became known, however, some women may have turned to them by choice in hope of faster deliveries. Their hopes stimulated a medical fashion. By about 1820 Dewees and Bard felt it necessary to condemn nervous young doctors for suc-

cumbing to the expectations of their patients and unnecessarily re-
sorting to forceps.[37]

How often physicians intervened with instruments is for the most
part a matter of conjecture. According to Bard of New York, instruments were in the hands of almost every practitioner by 1819 and were
commonly used. Professors of midwifery told students in strong terms
that ordinarily there was little need to interfere in labor with instruments or hands. Bard judged that "a fair opportunity of applying forceps will not occur to a rational practitioner in one of a thousand
cases."[38] Dewees, who thought the frequent use of forceps "really
alarming," estimated that he employed them in his own practice not
more than once in 350 cases, though he used them more often when
salvaging midwives' deliveries.[39] These rough estimates, and general
criticisms of the practice, suggest that trained physicians used instruments moderately, believing that "he who boasts of his skill and success in their application, is a very dangerous man."[40]

The formal education of American physicians and the development
of midwifery as a science, the desire of women for the best help in
childbirth, the utility of midwifery as a means of building a physician's practice, and ultimately the massive social changes associated with
urbanization explain why physicians assumed the ordinary practice of
midwifery among well-to-do urban women in the late eighteenth and
early nineteenth centuries. This development provides insight into the
changing condition of women in American society.

The development of obstetrics signified a partial rejection of the assumption that women had to suffer in childbirth and implied a new
social appreciation of women, as admonitions to women for forbear-
ance under the pains of labor turned to the desire to relieve their pain.
Thomas Denman explained that "The law of a religion founded on
principles of active benevolence, feelings of humanity, common interests of society, and special tenderness for women" demanded that men
search for a method by which women might be conducted safely
through childbirth.[41] American doctors used similar words to describe
their life's work, dwelling on woman's rightful and powerful claim to
their "highest concern."[42]

"Everything which affects the health, endangers the life, or produces the death of a female, especially a pregnant or parturient female

has stamped on it an importance that can be felt but not always expressed," Dr. John Rodgers told the members of the Medical Society of the State of New York as he began his presidential address in 1815. Aided by the grace that allows most orators to declaim on the inexpressible, Rodgers outlined the sources of woman's importance. Woman was not only valuable as "the companion of our lives, the solace of our cares, and resolver of our difficulties"; she also affected civil society. She "calmed the tumultuous passions of men," and, most compelling, she was "the chief agent in the education of children, and thereby forming the manners of the world. . . . Not one man in a thousand is fitted to teach children," proclaimed Rodgers, but woman, with her "cheerfulness, quick apprehensions, and better judgement of taste and propriety," was eminently qualified. This commanded the respect of men.[43]

While Rodgers thought that women's emotional and intellectual contribution to social life earned them the attention of obstetricians, Dewees felt that women deserved the compassion owed the weak. "How much then is she entitled to the sympathy of the other sex, and how much has it become their duty, by a careful investigation of her diseases, to discover the mode of relieving them!" he exclaimed, after unfavorably comparing woman's frail physique to that of man.[44]

The terms in which both doctors characterized women have come to be criticized as socially harmful female stereotypes, which unfortunately slights their historical meaning. Though their assumptions about women now appear false, these physicians had reached the innovative position that childbearing women deserved serious medical attention. However condescending some of their words sound today, and however imperfect their help may have been, physicians were concerned with the welfare of women. The American medical students who in 1812 drew a distinction between childbirth in primitive societies and their own perceived the implications of the change. In simple societies, "women are generally looked upon by their rugged lords as unworthy of any particular attention," and death or injury in childbirth is "not deemed a matter of any importance." Well-instructed assistants to women in childbirth were one sign of the value placed on women in civilized societies.[45]

The desire to relieve women in childbirth also signified a more liberal interpretation of scripture. At the University of Pennsylvania in 1804, Peter Miller, a medical student, modified the theological dictum that women must bear in sorrow. The anxieties of pregnancy and the anguish caused by the death of so many infants constituted sorrow enough for women, argued Miller. They did not need to be subjected to bodily pain as well.[46] Reiterating this argument, Dewees bluntly asked, "Why should the female alone incur the penalty of God?"[47] Dewees and Miller considered pain to be artificial, in that it was induced by civilization, and, Dewees thought, was "in part remediable." Their logic led them to analyze the physiology of childbirth and to devise techniques for relieving the pain of parturition.[48]

Whatever the origins of their sympathy for women, doctors maintained that it was requisite for good obstetrics. Channing recommended to his students at Boston Medical College the works of French women on midwifery because the women included "their particular sensations during their own confinement." By reading the French midwives La Motte and Baudiloque a man would "gain a great knowledge of the pains attendant on delivery."[49] Dr. Joseph Brevitt gave his readers detailed descriptions of the "tenderness, delicacy and sympathy" that ought to govern the actions of an obstetrician, and of the emotional rewards of delivering women. A woman in labor will cry, moan, and "accuse you of leaving her to suffer when she conceives it may be your power to remove it," Brevitt said with the authority of a man who had delivered 1,000 women. Be unruffled and compassionate, he advised; "remember that her mind is disordered by suffering." After delivery she will "perhaps verbally pronounce you (next to her God and father of her mercies) the saviour of the life of herself, and her beloved offspring," and you will "see her eyes glisten with a new, and perhaps till yet inexperienced delight of maternal love and affection." "If you are insensible" to these emotions, warned Brevitt, "drop your pursuit in this practice. You are not worthy of such superlative gratifications."[50]

If the development of obstetrics suggests the rise of a "special tenderness for women" on the part of men, it also meant that women's participation in medical practice was diminished and disparaged. A few American physicians instructed midwives or wrote manuals for them, but these efforts were private and sporadic, and had ceased by 1820.

The increasing professionalization of medicine, in the minds of the physicians who formed medical associations that set the standards of the field, left little room for female midwives, who lacked the prescribed measure of scientific training and professional identity.[51]

Though physicians ultimately dominated the practice of obstetrics, they disagreed among themselves about the place of midwives in the practice, sharing only the conviction that attendants at birth ought to be trained. Whether that attendant should ordinarily be a midwife or a physician—who almost without exception would be male—caused controversy for over a century in America. Initially dependent on midwives to call them to difficult labors, and only beginning to develop professional standards, physicians in the eighteenth century willingly taught midwives at least enough midwifery to know when a physician ought to be called for help.

British example in the eighteenth century suggested this approach. Male midwives directed the seven public lying-in hospitals opened in London during the century, but women managed the wards and studied there. The founders and directors thought, as did William Smellie, that midwives should be "perfectly well instructed" in the anatomy of the pelvis, skilled in examining women in labor and in delivering the placenta. She should, in sum, handle all routine deliveries but have recourse to a physician "when she finds herself at a loss."[52] Smellie urged men never to condemn openly a midwife's method of practice, because if "treated tenderly" midwives would be more apt to rely on doctors and consider them as friends rather than competitors. Smellie's advice sprang from the circumstances of his practice. He taught women, but his opinion that they "could hardly be supposed mistress" of all the qualifications of male midwives, and the fact that he did not include women in the count of his "regular" students, implies that he did not teach them how to use forceps.[53]

In Philadelphia, William Shippen initially invited midwives as well as medical students to attend his private courses in midwifery. His advertisement in the *Pennsylvania Gazette* in January 1765 related his experience assisting women in the country in difficult labors, "most of which was made so by the unskillful old women about them," and announced that he "thought it his duty to immediately begin" courses in midwifery "in order to instruct those women who have virtue enough to own their ignorance and apply for instructions, as well as those young gentlemen now engaged in the study of that useful and necessary branch of surgery." His private lessons included lectures on the use of instruments, "with necessary cautions against their dangerous and cruel use"; demonstrations on a dummy; and experience attending the labors of "a few poor women who otherwise might suffer for want of common necessities on these occasions," whom Shippen lodged. Shippen taught privately until after the Revolution, when he lectured only to the students at the University of Pennsylvania, who, of course, were male.[54]

At the turn of the century, Dr. Valentine Seaman conducted the only other known formal instruction of midwives. He was distressed by the ignorance of many midwives, yet was convinced that midwives ought to manage childbirth because, unlike physicians, they had time to wait out lingering labors, and, as women, they could deal easily with female patients. Seaman offered his private lectures and demonstrations at the New York Almshouse lying-in ward and in 1800 published them as the *Midwives Monitor and Mothers Mirror*.[55] A handful of other men wrote texts at least nominally directed to midwives between 1800 and 1810; some of these, like Seaman's, discussed the use of instruments.[56] In 1817 Dr. Thomas Ewell proposed that midwives be trained at a national school of midwifery in Washington, D.C., to be supported by a collection taken up by ministers. There is no evidence that Ewell's scheme, presented in his medical manual *Letters to Ladies*, ever provoked activity.[57]

Seaman, Ewell, and other authors of midwives' manuals presumed that if women mastered some of the fundamentals of obstetrics they would be desirable assistants in ordinary midwifery cases. Sharing this conviction, and tired of the many hours and night calls that midwifery demanded, two prominent Boston physicians, Dr. John Collins Warren and Dr. James Jackson, attempted about 1820 to transfer their practice to a midwife. Though Mrs. Alexander, a Scottish woman, held a British diploma in midwifery, and although, according to Dr. Warren, they "intended to relenquish only what belonged to ourselves, a great objection arose to this plan." Sensitive to the pressure from the other physicians of the Boston Medical Association, Drs. Warren and Jackson agreed to give up Mrs. Alexander.[58]

Their proposal had so aroused a colleague, probably Dr. Walter

Channing, that he presented his objections in a pamphlet, *Remarks on the Employment of Females as Practitioners in Midwifery*. Channing candidly admitted that midwives might deprive physicians of practice. However, "the only question which ought to be fairly considered," he wrote, "is, can the practice of midwifery be carried on with equal safety by female as by male practitioners?" Safety was the principal consideration, for by every other measure—woman's modesty, the efficient use of physicians' time, the small income derived from midwifery alone—women were the preferable practitioners.[59]

Channing decided that the possibility of danger that existed in every obstetrical case meant that men were the safest attendants. A routine delivery could turn swiftly into a medical emergency; and a hemorrhage, a convulsive fit, a retained placenta, or an inversion of the womb would require the "prompt and judicious treatment" of a physician. The man called "at the moment of hurry and danger" was denied the opportunity to stem the problem in its early stages and lacked the insights derived from long-term care of the patient. In other cases, the mother might suffer from a disorder unrelated to the reproductive system, which only a physician could discriminate and treat. Labor was not simply a mechanical process, but affected the entire system. No one, Channing maintained, could completely understand the management of labor who did not understand "thoroughly the profession of medicine as a whole."[60]

Implementation of Channing's principle would have totally excluded women from midwifery, because no one favored professional medical education for women. It was generally assumed that they could not easily master the necessary languages, mathematics, and chemistry or withstand the trials of dissecting room and hospital. Channing emphasized that women's moral character disqualified them for medical practice. "Their feelings of sympathy are too powerful for the cool exercise of judgement" in medical emergencies, he wrote. "They do not have the power of action, nor the active power of mind which is essential to the practice of the surgeon."[61]

Though Channing successfully disparaged midwives, he managed to do it without assuming a scornful tone. This was an achievement of sorts, since most physicians who wrote on the subject invariably modified the word "midwife" with the word "ignorant." Bard contrasted the physician, a "candid and unprejudiced young man," with "anxious" patients, "mistaken" friends, and "common" midwives. When all the women about him became hysterical, he retained "firmness and self-possession." Dewees criticized the practices of midwives as unscientific and therefore foolish. Walking about during the first stages of labor was a "preposterous custom" that "should be peremptorily forbidden." The tying and dressing of the umbilical cord was "now a process of great simplicity among the more enlightened of the community," whereas the old ceremony had been produced by "ignorance and craft." The idea that a woman needed spirits and nourishing food such as meat after delivery was a "vulgar error"; she needed an invalid's bland diet of tea, oatmeal, and tapioca for five days after giving birth.[62]

Other physicians did not limit themselves to critical adjectives. Dr. William Baker, Jr., a proud member of the "Medical and Chirurgical Faculty of Maryland," composed an attack on midwives, "the ignorant old women, who can be guided by nothing but vague experience and false analogy." Baker was confident that "every gentleman of the profession must have frequent occasions to lament the obstinacy of erroneous custom, and the sad effects of female quackery, in cases of labor." "Daily experience proves," he wrote in 1810, how many women "fall victims to improper management of midwives" and how necessary was the care of a physician throughout pregnancy and parturition.[63] Through extremes of argument and language, Baker sought to prove that midwives—mere female quacks—were dangerous alternatives to physicians.

Midwives responded only in a limited way to criticism and competition from physicians. They began advertising in newspapers in the decade before the Revolution, and their notices stressed that the subscriber was trained in her art by "first practitioners in midwifery" or by "celebrated professors" and would answer any call immediately. At least one midwife advertised in 1789 that she "had the advantage" of the instruction of Dr. Shippen of Philadelphia.[64] Midwife M. Hartley of New York City announced her record of a successful London practice but considered that her "great Tenderness and Delicacy, to her own Sex, will be a better Recommendation than any thing She might say in her own Behalf."[65]

Collaboration and conflict took place as midwives and doctors encountered each other more frequently in the lying-in room. The dimensions of this contact are sketched out in the diary of midwife Martha Ballard, who practiced in the agricultural community of Augusta, Maine, from 1785 to 1812. Ballard, who delivered 996 women with only 4 recorded fatalities, freely consulted doctors in difficult cases. Doctors, in turn, borrowed herbal medicines from her, copied her records of births and deaths, and sent her patients; one trusted her to deliver his wife. This professional relationship included an invitation to "the Decexion of Rachel Savage," which, Ballard recorded, twelve doctors and three midwives attended.[66] Yet, at times, the association between doctor and midwife became strained, as it did when Dr. Cony raged at Ballard for meddling by giving her opinion of a disease "and said this was one of the many instances I had done so." Midwife Ballard hoped that "those who I am called to meet with" would defend her, but she confronted her accusers without satisfaction and concluded, "this is a world of tryale."[67]

Other American midwives would have understood Ballard's dismay when her activities were challenged by a physician. Denied formal medical training, midwives of the early nineteenth century could not claim any other professional or legal status. Unlike Great Britain, the United States had no extensive record of licensing laws or oaths defining the practice of midwifery. Nor were there any vocal groups of midwives who, conscious of their tradition of practice, trained by physicians, or associated with lying-in hospitals, were able to defend themselves against competition. Though men assumed care of well-to-do women in Britain, midwives who served the lower classes had some access to education.[68] American midwives ceased practice among urban women of social rank with few words uttered in their support.

The success of the physicians produced its own problems. The doctor's sex affected the relationships between women and their attendants in childbirth and transformed the atmosphere of the lying-in room. In his advice to his male students Dewees acknowledged that summoning a man to assist in childbed "cost females a severe struggle."[69] Other doctors knew that even the ordinary gynecologic services of a physician occasioned embarrassment and violated woman's "natural delicacy of feeling."[70] Every sensitive woman felt "deeply humiliated"

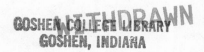

at the least bodily exposure, which forced doctors to treat vaginal disorders without ever seeing the diseased parts.[71] Doctors recognized an almost universal repugnance on the part of women to male assistance in time of labor.[72] Because of "whim or false delicacy" women often refused to call a man until their condition had become critical.[73] It is unlikely that physicians exaggerated these observations, although there is little testimony from women themselves about their childbed experience in the early nineteenth century.

The uneasiness of women who were treated by men was sometimes shared by their husbands. In 1772 the *Virginia Gazette* printed a denunciation of male midwifery as immoral. The author, probably an Englishman, attributed many cases of adultery in England to the custom of employing men at deliveries. Even in labor a woman enjoyed intervals of ease, and these, he thought, were the moments when the doctor infringed on the privileges of the husband. It would be a matter of utmost indifference to him "whether my wife had spent the night in a bagnio, or an hour of the forenoon locked up with a man midwife in her dressing room."[74] These arguments were frequently and seriously raised in England during the eighteenth century.[75] They may seem ludicrous, but at least one American man of Dr. Ewell's acquaintance suffered emotional conflict over hiring a male midwife. He sent for a physician to help his wife in her labor, yet "very solemnly he declared to the doctor, he would demolish him if he touched or looked at his wife."[76]

Physicians dealt with the embarrassment of patients and the suspicions of husbands by observing the drawing room behavior of "well-bred gentlemen." Dewees told his students to "endeavour by a general and well chosen conversation, to divert the patient's mind from the purpose of your visit."[77] All questions of a delicate nature were to be communicated through a third party, perhaps the only other person in the room, either a nurse or an elderly friend or relative. The professional man was advised "never to seem to know anything about the parts of generation, further than that there is an orifice near the rectum leading to an os."[78]

Physicians did not perform vaginal examinations unless it was absolutely necessary to do so, and they often had to cajole women into permitting an examination. Nothing could be more shocking to a woman, Shippen lectured his students, "than for a young man the moment he enters the Chamber to ask for Pomatum and proceed to examine the uterus."[79] Doctors waited until a labor pain clutched their patients and then suggested an examination by calling it "taking a pain." The light in the room was dimmed by closing the shutters during the day and covering the lamps at night. During examination and delivery the patient lay completely covered in her bed, a posture more modest, if less comfortable, than squatting on a pallet or a birth stool. If a physician used forceps, he had to manipulate them under the covers, using his free hand as a guide.[80] On this point, doctors who read Thomas Denman's *Obstetrical Remembrancer* were reminded that "Degorges, one of the best obstetricians of his time, was blind."[81]

The crowd of supportive friends and family disappeared with the arrival of the doctor. The physician guarded against too many attendants; "where there are women, they must talk."[82] The presence of many other women might increase the doctor's nervousness, and they certainly did not help the woman in labor, who ought to rest and remain quiet. Medical men interpreted women's talk of other experiences with childbirth as mere gossip about difficult and dangerous labor, which ought to be stopped lest it disturb the patient.[83] Especially distracting were the bawdy stories visitors told, expecting the physician to laugh, too. Medical professors recommended serious demeanor, warning that levity would lower the patient's opinion of the physician.[84]

Far from providing the consolation of a friend, the physician was often a stranger who needed to "get a little acquainted" with his patient. One medical text went so far as to coach him in a series of conversational icebreakers about children and the weather.[85] Nor did the physician offer the reassurance of his continual presence. If they tarried too long in the room, Channing informed his students, their patient would suffer a distended bladder, as women disliked urinating before the physician.[86] Dewees added that by remaining in the "sick room" as little as was consistent with duty, doctors would "apparently abridge" the period of waiting.[87] When experience had taught him to anticipate the progress of labor, the physician might also use the waiting time more profitably and leave the house for short periods to conduct other business.[88]

Etiquette and prudery in the lying-in chamber affected medical care. Physicians were frustrated by their inability to examine their patients thoroughly, for they knew full well that learning midwifery from a book was like learning to build a ship without touching wood.[89] Examinations were inadequate, and the dangers of manipulating instruments without benefit of sight were tremendous. Dewees cautioned his students to take great care before pulling the forceps that "no part of the mother is included in the locking of the blades. This accident is frequent."[90] Accidental mutilation of infants was also reported, as the navel string had to be cut under the covers. Lecturers passed on the story of the incautious doctor who included the penis of an infant within the blades of his scissors.[91]

In view of such dangers, the conflict between social values and medical practice is striking. The expansion of medical knowledge brought men and women face to face with social taboos in family life.[92] They had to ask themselves the question: Who should watch a woman give birth? For centuries the answer had unhesitatingly been female relatives and friends and the midwife. The science of obstetrics, developing in the eighteenth century, changed the answer. Though socially women might be the most acceptable assistants at delivery, men were potentially more useful. Americans came to think that, as Thomas Jefferson advised his pregnant daughter in 1803, "The material thing is to have scientific aid in readiness, that if anything uncommon takes place, it may be redressed on the spot."[93]

In consequence of the attendance of male physicians, by 1825 childbirth was ceasing to be an open ceremony for some American women. Though birth still took place at home, and though friends and relatives still lent a helping hand, visiting women no longer dominated the activities of the lying-in room. The physician limited visitors because they hindered proper medical care, but the process of birth was also concealed because it embarrassed both patient and physician.

Between 1760 and 1825 childbirth was thus transformed from an open affair to a restricted one. As one consequence of the development of obstetrics as a legitimate branch of medicine, male physicians began replacing midwives. They began to reduce childbirth to a scientifically managed event and deprived it of its folk aspects. Strengthened by the professionalization of the field, these physicians responded to the hopes of women in Philadelphia, New York, and Boston for safe delivery. Although they helped some pregnant women, they hurt midwives, who were shut out of an area of medicine that had been traditionally their domain. All these innovations took place in the large urban centers, in response to distinctly urban phenomena. They reflected the increasing privatization of family life, and they foreshadowed mid-nineteenth-century attitudes toward childbirth, mothers, and women.

CHAPTER 3

Mothers and Children in the Colonial Years

When she composed her feminist manifesto *Women and Economics*, Charlotte Perkins Gilman thought that the subject of motherhood needed to be approached with special mental preparation. In 1898, wrote Gilman, a man might "question the purposes and methods of his God with less danger of outcry against him than if he dare to question the purposes and methods of his mother." She perceived an American matriolatry "so deep-seated, wide-spread, and long-established as to be dominant in every class of minds."[1]

Gilman's ridicule of modern mother worship reveals how well she withstood popular sentimental conventions. "The dying soldier on the battlefield thinks of his mother, longs for her, not his father," she wrote, evoking the Civil War ballad "Just Before the Battle, Mother," and continued bitingly, "The traveler and exile dreams of his mother's care, his mother's doughnuts."[2] The pathos of the popular story in the nineteenth century was bringing the prodigal back to his mother, not to his father. What Gilman truly exaggerated was the age of this matriolatry. It was not an ancient phenomenon but had grown almost entirely within the nineteenth century.

Beginning in the middle of the eighteenth century, some Americans slowly began to defer the pattern of family life into the small, emotionally intense units familiar to us. Though exceptions abound among different social classes, ethnic groups, and geographic regions, it is on the whole accurate to say that two things came to characterize family life in the complex urban, industrial, commercial, and secular societies that developed in western Europe and America. In the modern family the mother is regarded socially as the most important parent, and a substantial part of family life focuses on childrearing. Ideally, in modern families, women were supposed to remain in the home and devote themselves to the care of children; or, as Gilman put it, women were "saved from direct economic activity" so they could "concentrate all their energies on the beautiful work of motherhood."[3]

This ideal of "spiritualized motherhood," which has become a source of profound conflict in a nation where over half of all married women are employed outside the home, is actually a relatively recent creation. Colonial women were much more concerned with childbearing than with childrearing. The daily tasks of managing their homes left them little time for worrying about their children's psychological development, and both economic necessity and religious doctrine encouraged children to grow up quickly. During the late eighteenth and early nineteenth centuries, however, subtle changes took place that elevated women's role as mothers into a sacred calling. At the same time, the birthrate in most parts of the United States began to decline. As childbirth became less frequent for American women, child nurture became their all-absorbing task.

Although this emphasis on motherhood has been decried in modern times as an effort to restrict woman's activities outside the home, it is important to realize that, historically, the new social ideal was only superficially conservative. The mother worship of the nineteenth century represented a new appreciation of woman's moral and intellectual capacities, as well as an accommodation to new forms of economic life.

Ultimately, the new ideals of motherhood and new assumptions about women affected childbearing practices as well. Sentimental reverence for motherhood provided a climate in which women legitimately could limit the size of their families, physicians could justify scientific changes in the management of pregnancy and birth, and social reformers could press for public maternal health programs.

The radical aspects of mother worship are clearer when we compare the lives of colonial and nineteenth-century women, though to make such a comparison is a step into the cross fire of a historian's controversy. The history of colonial women has become a battleground for academics preoccupied with judging the impact of industrialization and colonization on Americans; indeed, the status of colonial woman is debated more extensively now than it ever was in the seventeenth and eighteenth centuries.

The general lack of recorded native discourse on or by colonial women is, in itself, a clue that the years before the late eighteenth century were not a golden age for women. Neither immigration to the New World nor the work patterns of a preindustrial society resulted in independence for colonial women, who lived, for the most part, crippled by patriarchally oriented law, economy, and social conventions. While it is true that the household manufactures of colonial women were an "integral part of the early political economy of the colonies," as Elizabeth Dexter put it in her influential history, there is little evidence to support her conclusion that colonial craftswomen, weavers, artisans, and shopkeepers pursued their businesses "outside the limited home circle," in "a legal and social atmosphere of entire freedom" that disappeared with the industrialization of America.[4] Other historians have considered women's status as a dimension of the American colonial and frontier experience, arguing that because of woman's value as a scarce commodity on the frontier and simplified legal practices in the colonies, colonial courts tended to treat women as equals before the law.[5] However, analysis of the legal system in Pennsylvania shows that the conditions of colonial life did not create a new liberal legal climate for married women.[6] Despite early accommodations to the colonial setting and preindustrial labor patterns, most women, of all classes, did not enjoy occupational prestige or social and legal equality with men. The assumptions that women were subordinate to men and that their chief occupation was bearing children and managing households persisted.

The literature of advice on social relations read or written by colonials outlined a hierarchy in which men managed the world and women managed the house. English guides circulated throughout the colonies reminded women that to be happy with a husband they must "first lay it down for a Foundation in general, that there is Inequality in the sexes."[7] Even New England Puritans, who emphasized the reciprocal rights and duties of husband and wife and urged spouses to practice mutual love and respect, maintained that husbands were "ever to be esteemed the superior," saying that when a wife "cannot with calm Reasons convince him of Inexpediencies, she submits her will and Sense to his."[8] The faithful wife did not stray "too much from home" upon concerns that were perhaps "unaccountable" to her husband. Her work lay in the house, and if her husband were asked where she was, he should be able to answer, as Abraham did, "My wife is in the tent."[9]

To be sure, didactic literature expresses model rather than actual behavior, and there are examples enough to show that some women mastered both husbands and businesses.[10] In the broad context, however, social practice mimicked prescriptions. The women who ran farm households certainly were not the pretty gentlewomen of advice literature, but most of them worked, as the ladies' books described woman's life, at home in the service of their husbands and family.

Colonial housekeeping demanded continual labor. Wealth or geography might relieve women of some work—many hired servants, and city living limited farming chores to kitchen gardens—but the overwhelming majority of women lived on small- to middle-sized farms. In addition to the feminine chores of cooking, cleaning, and childcare, farm women manufactured most textiles and preserved all the food for their families. An advertisement for a woman to manage "The female concerns of a country business," which appeared in the *Pennsylvania Packet* during 1780, describes in abbreviated form the work of an ordinary farm wife who spent her days "raising small stock, dairying, marketing, combing, carding, spinning, knitting, sewing, pickling, preserving, etc. and the occasional instruction of two young ladies." The et cetera concealed a multitude of heavy and monotonous daily tasks, such as tending a vegetable garden, hauling wood and water to the kitchen, and cooking over an open fire. Only the slow cycle of the seasons varied the work, breaking the year into times of growing, gathering, and preserving the harvest.[11]

Some women gained satisfaction in knowing that their work contributed directly to the survival of their families, but many of the women who managed to keep a journal of their activities described their boredom, frustration, and exhaustion. "Full of freting discontent dirty and miserabel both yesterday and today," wrote Mary Cooper of Long Island after two weeks of soap- and candlemaking that followed the hog butchering in December 1769.[12]

Women pursued a variety of trades, but almost all their employments were related to household work. Textile manufacture, the most important craft of almost all women, was traditionally a female task carried on in the home.[13] The tavernkeeping and shopkeeping of urban women also were extensions of domestic duties, not generally independent enterprises.

Married tradeswomen almost invariably worked in association with their husbands. This domestic, shared enterprise originated in the household organization of manufacturing and merchandising as well as in the legal disabilities of married women. The wife of an artisan usually kept house in or beside his workplace and easily became involved with his work. Benjamin Franklin succinctly described this situation in his Philadelphia house and printing shop when he recalled that, about 1730, Deborah Franklin "assisted me cheerfully in my business, folding and stitching pamphlets, tending shop, purchasing old linen rags for the paper-makers, etc., etc."[14] This form of feminine labor was not uniquely American, a product of necessity in the labor-short colonies; European artisans and tradesmen commonly were assisted by their wives, and widows carried on businesses after their husbands' deaths.[15]

Only single women possessed the unquestionable legal right to conduct businesses independently. Married women, whose legal existence was subsumed under their husbands', could not make contracts to trade in their own names. The detailed antenuptial contract that Elizabeth Murray Smith negotiated with her third husband in 1771 illustrates the maneuvers that were necessary if a married woman were to do business. In order to preserve her power to buy and sell property, protect her own income, and retain her right to make a valid will, this Boston businesswoman had to get an explicit document in which her future husband agreed to keep their property separate. In essence, he promised to be her agent, signing whatever contracts she wanted him to, without questioning her judgment or taking the money she might earn.[16]

Shrewd and wealthy, Elizabeth Murray Smith was an unusual

woman who confidently directed her farms and dry-goods trade by circumventing her legal status as a married woman. Most women worked on a family farm or business but did not share either the control or the profits of such enterprises. Few of them grasped the broader aspects of the family economy. The Loyalist women from all ranks who filed reparations petitions with the British government after the Revolution were familiar with the day-to-day operations of their farms and businesses but lacked knowledge of the total assets as well as of the structure of the enterprises.[17] For the most part, their work had been part of their household labor.

However, that seventeenth- and eighteenth-century women lived private, housebound lives does not mean that their domestic lives resembled those of twentieth-century housewives. Caring for young children is the most important domestic responsibility of twentieth-century women; for women of the seventeenth and eighteenth centuries, the task of housekeeping, with all the manufacturing that it involved, mattered more than childrearing. Though colonial women spent more of their lives bearing and nursing children, they devoted less attention to rearing them. As Laurel Thatcher Ulrich put it in her book on colonial New England women, "Mothering in early New England was extensive rather than intensive."[18] The mistress of a household, farm, or business could not absorb herself in childcare, nor was she expected to. Father, siblings, other relatives, servants, or the masters to whom the child might be apprenticed shared the supervision and training of a child with its mother.

The general lack of sentiment attached to the tasks of childrearing in the seventeenth and early eighteenth centuries is particularly striking from our distance. Parents tried to cultivate respect and obedience, rather than affection, from their children, and mothers who were devoted to their infants chided themselves for their indulgence. No social critics, no legal or religious authorities claimed, as they would extravagantly in the coming centuries, that mothers were the "most powerful influence in the formation of the character of man" or said that "the best pleasures of a woman's life are found in the faithful discharge of her maternal duties."[19] Only recently has being a mother ideally meant emotional absorption in the lives of her children.

Far from exalting the relationship between mother and child,

Americans assigned it a modest rank in the hierarchy of family relationships and feminine responsibilities. Their literature on family life
generally considers the parental, rather than the maternal, role in
childrearing; often the advice is addressed to literate "Syrs."[20] The
masculine pronoun is the one small sign of the patriarchal cast of family life. Law and custom confirmed that the father ought to govern his
family as a head of state governed his subjects. Women, as we have
seen, had comparatively little power in the family or the state, and
children had less.

The status of women and children in the family has changed pro-
foundly during the last 200 years, at the expense of paternal power.
Given new social and economic contexts, we have redefined the functions of the family, placing a high value on emotional bonds between
mother and child. We have redistributed power among members of
the family, even in the narrowest legal sense, restricting the power of
fathers, enlarging that of mothers, and making the power of both sub-
servient to the welfare of children.

In legal terms the Anglo-American family was, as Blackstone observed in 1768, "the empire of the father." Under common law, the
father had almost unlimited rights to the custody, control, and services of his children, whereas the mother, Blackstone wrote tersely,
was "entitled to no power, but only to reverence and respect." The
primacy of fathers' rights extended even in cases when neglect or bru-
tality forced women to separate from their husbands, or when the
welfare of young children might be served more suitably by leaving
them in their mothers' care. A father also had the privilege of dele-
gating his paternal rights to a guardian, rather than letting them fall
to his spouse after his death. The colonial courts rarely overruled fathers'
rights. Judges who considered child custody cases in the years after
the Revolution declared that there was no precedent for depriving fathers
of their children.[21]

Patterns of property ownership strengthened paternal authority.
Where fathers controlled the disposition of land, as they did in stable
agricultural towns such as Andover and Hingham, Massachusetts,
during the seventeenth century, sons remained economically dependent on them well into maturity, just as they did in European farming
communities. A father who was reluctant to transfer control of his

property to his sons delayed their marriages and tied them to his household. Conversely, the inability of married women to control their earnings or property without special provision materially affected their claims on their children. In their wills, fathers assigned children to male guardians rather than to their mothers in order to protect their estates from possible abuse by a stepfather. A woman could not defend their property, since her power would disappear on remarriage.[22]

Theology supported a patriarchy entrenched legally and economically. The title of Benjamin Wadsworth's book *The Well-Ordered Family: or, Relative Duties*, introduces his themes. Discipline and duty, he argues, are the firmest foundations of family life. Wadsworth assumed that social order originates in strong family government, and his assumption, as well as the hierarchical pattern of family organization that he outlined, was common in Anglo-American literature of family life. The family, we read, is a model of the larger commonwealth, its members linked by bonds of authority and subjection. Parents and children of a biological family, as well as servants who shared the household, owed duties and deference to each other according to their relative age, sex, and condition of servitude. Children and servants, who were "in some sort likewise our children," stood in the lowest rank; then, as we have seen, wife and mother, and at the head, the "Owner of a Family," who was to "faithfully Command and Manage those that belong unto him."[23]

This scheme of family relationships, supported by scripture, was not novel in western Europe, but a specifically Protestant interpretation initially emphasized paternal power in the family. The Protestant reforms reduced the authority of priests and elevated that of laymen, who were charged with leading household devotions. Fathers conducted daily prayers, Bible readings, and catechism lessons. Conscientious men also observed their children at play, searching games for moral lessons that later might be pointed out to the young, and assigned meditations to be written in copybooks.[24] Thus, domestic spiritual exercises reinforced the moral authority of Anglican and Puritan fathers.

Puritan parents explicitly equated a child's service to them with service to God, on the theory that until a child obeyed its father it could never obey God. Believing that children were "slaves of Divels," much closer to original sin than disciplined adults, Puritans worked to break the wills of their children during the first years of their lives. Children acquired an understanding of their Christian duty slowly, by pain, chastisement, and progressive exercise of reason. Whipping, constant reminders of damnation, and strict schedules—all administered in the name of eternal salvation—subjugated children to parental will. Although fathers left us most of the descriptions of this process, and male theologians elaborated on the intellectual justification for harsh discipline, women fearing for the souls of their children also inflicted harsh physical correction on their children. Esther Burr, for example, began to govern her daughter Sally while she was in her cradle, whipping her once "on Old Adams account" before she was ten months old.[25]

Mothers shared the Christian duty to teach children religious principles, as well as the legal obligation to govern and nurture them, but very little advice was addressed to women in the literature on family life. Advice on their special responsibilities appears almost parenthetically, incorporated into chapters on "House, Family and Children." In 1699, Cotton Mather, the most frequently published American author between 1689 and 1740, injected one aside on the subject into his treatise on family life: "And let it be Remembered, That the Fathers are not the only Parents obliged thus to pursue the Salvation of their Children."[26] The few words in advice literature addressed to women on their maternal duties counseled them to care for themselves in pregnancy and to suckle their infants but treated childrearing as a cooperative effort, or left only the education of girls to the mother as her proper jurisdiction.[27]

The literature explicitly discouraged women from excessive emotional attachment to their children. Children, ministers warned, were not the creations or possessions of mothers. The ideal mother "look'd upon her Children as meer Loans from God, which he may call for when he please." Knowing that her children were God's, she did not "roar like a Beast and howl I cannot bear it" if they died. And, as a parent, she did not take credit if they were "perfect"; nor did she "give them her heart," which belonged to God.[28] Similar moderation marks the advice of a secular man, who told women that they might love their children "without living in the Nursery" and take competent care of them without making them the subject of all their conversations.[29]

Of course, these warnings against emotional attachment to children imply that some women did treat their children affectionately. Unfortunately, we have few words on the matter from women until about 1750. Not many women described their family life between Anne Bradstreet, who wrote her domestic poems in the middle of the seventeenth century, and Eliza Pinckney, who wrote fondly of the "thousand beauties" of her baby boy Charles 100 years later.[30] The funeral sermons that ministers delivered for their own mothers early in the eighteenth century evoke images of maternal tenderness and devotion. Cotton Mather compared the consolation of God with that given by mothers, though God's consolations were "beyond what the most affectionate mother on Earth" could give. Both fed and clothed their children, preserved them from harm, and let them "know that it is a Pleasure unto them to see us." Thomas Foxcroft remembered his mother as a woman "easy and soft, yet without weakness," who used her "authority without severity," was "strict without ill nature," and who was always "so tenderly careful" of her children.[31]

Yet these sermons are remarkable because they also reveal inhibitions about maternal affection. It was only "sometimes the happiness of a mother" to have sons who paid her homage in the manner of Foxcroft and Mather. "For the most part," Mather had written elsewhere, he saw in men "Readiness to Slight their Mothers."[32] When there was affection, as in the case of the two ministers, that feeling was tempered by fears that it was inappropriate to give a mother too much "seat in our Hearts," as Mather put it. Foxcroft thought that a mother's death could be God's jealous punishment of children to "over-rate and over-love" their parent. He began his funeral oration with a lengthy series of reasons justifying his mourning and, like Mather, praised his mother as a model Christian more than as a model woman. Foxcroft appended to his sermon a spiritual biography of his mother, the better to emphasize the important lessons of her life, and Mather concluded his sermon with the threat that biological and emotional ties would mean nothing to a Christian mother if her children were ungodly. Should they err, she would be, not their comforter, but their "grievous Accuser."[33]

Ambivalence marks the memorials that these Puritan sons wrote about their mothers, as it also marked the way most early modern parents thought and felt about their children.[34] Some of the intellectual sources of ambivalence appear in the writings of men and women—usually evangelical Protestants—who speculated on the nature of children. While they saw that some children presented innocent and appealing faces to the world, the sweetness, they decided, was only apparent. Even the very best children were corrupt with Adam's sin. Samuel Willard's description of children as "innocent vipers" captures the ambivalence of the Puritan father toward his child.[35] Parental affection could not prevent early discipline, control, and education of the children. Children no sooner stepped than they strayed, no sooner lisped than they lied, wrote Cotton Mather, encouraging parents to chastise their children, however young.[36]

Parents of gentler religious views regarded their children more indulgently. When they looked at their small children, they were more likely to see a "copy of Adam before he tasted of Eve or the Apple" and to consider education a process of bending, rather than breaking, childish wills.[37] However, securing obedience from their children preoccupied the colonial parents who have left us records of their thoughts on childrearing, and all consciously rejected the "foolish fondness of seeming tenderness" toward children because it undermined parental authority.[38] Instilling discipline in their children concerned mothers as well as fathers. Women like Sally Logan Fisher promised themselves, as well as their husbands, that they would not indulge their children "in every thing their little fancys crave, but early . . . teach them a strict lesson of Obedience, knowing they will in the end be much happier."[39]

These are the words of a conscientious, articulate parent. The Fishers, like the Sewalls, Mathers, and Adamses, tried to maintain a balance between parental affection and parental authority; their writings show us that they lived with the consequent tensions. However, the meager public records suggest that inarticulate parents, those with less education and wealth, regarded their children with less concern. Among the parents who filed for divorce in eighteenth-century Massachusetts courts, for example, the cultural ambivalence about children drifted into indifference. Almost all the petitioners spoke of their children as economic quantities, and many clearly treated them in a cavalier, even abusive way. Even more revealing than accounts of child beating is children's testimony about their parents' adulteries. Clearly, their parents were not concerned with preserving the supposed innocence of their children.[40]

What we know of colonial childrearing practices indicates that a child's place in the network of family and community was, like its stature, little and low. Parents often regarded their children chiefly as economic assets, not primarily as a source of emotional satisfaction. Indeed, the responsibility for a child's development might fall on masters, siblings, and neighbors as much as on parents. The diffusion of childcare into the community represents one form of parental detachment from children. Other practices demonstrate that parents treated children, especially infants, impersonally.

When parents name a child, they announce the presence of a new person in the world. Colonial parents delayed recognizing their children as individuals, frequently referring to their infants as "it," "the little stranger," or "the baby."[41] When little strangers became familiar, parents began to call them by their names that identified their sex and place in the family. Usually a child's first name was not unique. New England parents named children after themselves, grandparents, aunts, and uncles, thereby stressing the generational continuity of the family rather than the individuality of each child. It was also the custom in America through the middle of the eighteenth century, as it was in England, to name children after dead siblings, so that in one family three sons might bear the name John. They would also give several living children the same name to increase the chances that the patronymic, if not all the children, would survive.[42]

Other childrearing practices diminished the individuality of young children, as well as separating them from their mothers. Almost immediately after birth children were transformed into little bundles by the mummylike wrapping of swaddling clothes, which prevented motion and limited skin contact with mothers. And wet nurses commonly suckled infants, sometimes removing their charges to their own homes.

Swaddling of infants, an ancient practice, was customary in England through the mid-eighteenth century. Until then, infants ordinarily were wound in a broad strip of linen, ostensibly to prevent them from distorting their soft bones by motion. After four months the child's arms would be freed, but for the first year its chest, belly, and legs were bound. While there are no descriptions of swaddling in seventeenth-century America, there are occasional entries of "swathing bands" in inventories, and it seems unlikely that colonial women abandoned a universal British custom in the seventeenth century only to resume it in the eighteenth. Like their British sisters, American women encased their children in linen, converting their infants into packages, easy to carry about or even hang on a peg on a wall. Undeniably convenient for adults, swaddling, in the words of critic Dr. William Cadogan, extinguished children's "liberty," denying them the power to "act and exert themselves." The individuality of children, expressed in the grasping of tiny hands and the kicking of small feet, disappeared under bands of linen. Swaddling made it easier to consider babies objects rather than people.[43]

Nearly all American children nursed at the breast, though not necessarily that of their mother. Wet nurses, lactating women hired to suckle children, often nursed infants. Though widespread in Europe, it is difficult to assess how prevalent the practice of wet-nursing was in seventeenth-century America. It appears to have been acceptable to hire wet nurses for the first weeks of an infant's life; the prominent Boston families of the Mathers and the Sewalls routinely employed them. Hiring a nurse was justified while the mother recovered from her lying-in, if she were sick, had scanty milk, or was too weak to nurse. However, mothers were subject to criticism if they refused to nurse merely because of laziness or fastidiousness.[44]

In the eighteenth century wet-nursing seems to have remained common. Breast milk, judges one historian of colonial pediatrics, was the most frequently advertised commodity in American newspapers. During the second half of the century nearly every newspaper contained the advertisements of women who would nurse infants in the salubrious air of their country homes, or who would move in with the infant's family. Most urban nurses probably did not even need to advertise. Philadelphian Elizabeth Drinker found it easy in 1781 to arrange for "the Shoemakers wife next door to come in 4 or 5 times a Day" to nurse her child, and southern women, particularly those of plantation gentry in Virginia and the Carolinas, gave their infants to slave nurses— a custom that shocked strangers.[45]

Mothers who passed their infants to wet nurses severed early the physiological bonds with their children. They were not forced to answer infants' cries for nourishment. They also did not experience the relief of having distended breasts drained or the erotic stimulation that nursing infants give to their mothers. Extreme evidence of the sympathy that could be aroused between nurse and child appears in the accounts of southern white children who grieved when their black nurses were whipped.[46]

Accepted practices of childcare, swaddling, and wet-nursing fostered detachment of mothers from infants. Other arrangements discouraged maternal attachments to older children and suggest that colonials placed little value on a close association between mother and child. In large colonial households grandparents, older siblings, and servants shared the feeding and supervision of children, and some children above the age of seven were bound outside their families as apprentices and servants.

If colonial families were not as large as early historians fancied them, they were, nonetheless, big and extended by our standards. Several remarkable features of colonial family structure helped shape the pattern of childrearing. Because colonial women bore children throughout their fertile years, there was likely to be a considerable range of ages among the children of any family. Young men and women of twenty lived in the same house as their toddling brothers and sisters, and they commonly supervised the youngsters. Another generation of watchful relatives, widowed grandparents, also shared the residence and chores of childrearing.[47] Frequently, servants or boarders augmented the number of blood relations living together, helping to bring the household size in Massachusetts, one state for which we have statistics, to an average of seven in 1764, larger by one person than the average family.[48] In some well-to-do northern families, servants took almost complete routine care of children, as did slaves in the South; in modest households servants were parental auxiliaries.[49] Thus, the permutations of age, generation, and bondage in colonial households meant that most children received care from people other than their mothers.

Apprenticeship and indenture, which served a variety of economic and educational purposes in the colonies, also increased the distance between mothers and children. In America, plagued by labor short-age, the trade education provided by apprenticeship was more impor-tant than its effect in controlling the skilled labor market, which en-couraged the system in Europe. Throughout the colonies parents voluntarily apprenticed youths of ten to fourteen years, and occasion-ally children as young as six or seven, to live with masters who were obliged to teach them trades and oversee their elementary education; but American apprenticeships tended to be shorter than European ones, which pushed journeymen sooner into the market.[50]

Civil authorities bound out poor and rejected children under similar terms, and the records of compulsory indenture and apprenticeship of these wards of the community spell out a few of the reasons why chil-dren were bound out. Colonials assumed that children should begin to work at an early age. Tending cows, sorting and carding wool, weaving strips of tape for clothing were tasks for seven-year-olds in the colonies, and adults knew that the children who performed them learned crafts, contributed to their upkeep, and saved themselves from the sin of idleness. Overseers of the poor, concerned with preventing children from becoming public charges, traded on the acceptability and profitability of child labor; the commercial importance of child labor emerged early in Virginia, where the governors arranged shipments of London waifs to serve in the New World.[51]

Parents may have had other reasons, too, for voluntarily apprentic-ing their children. Some New England parents bound out their chil-dren even when there was no apparent educational or economic ad-vantage in doing so, an action that is especially puzzling in the case of girls bound out to learn housekeeping in families of equivalent social rank. Edmund Morgan speculates that Puritan parents made these ap-prenticeships because they were afraid of spoiling their own children. They deemed the separation of parent and child salutary and gave their children to people who would discipline them impartially.[52]

Whatever the causes—economic, pedagogical, or psychological—that led parents to sign apprenticeship papers, the consequence was the same. Children went to live with their masters and might see their parents rarely. They received vocational training in a family but not in their own families. Child apprenticeship, common at all levels of colonial society, indicates that it was acceptable and perhaps, in the case of the

Puritans, even considered desirable to separate mothers and children.

It is impossible to measure precisely how many colonial children worked at apprenticeships. The estimates for two New England towns in the seventeenth century range widely; perhaps from 10 to 30 percent of the children in Plymouth and Bristol spent some part of their childhood outside the parental roof.[53] Likewise, we cannot know precisely how many infants were swaddled or how many were put out to nurse. It is the multiplicity of childrearing practices separating mothers and children, taken together with the cautions in advice literature, the provisions of the law, and the meager descriptions of child life in personal records, which tell us that close maternal ties were not of paramount importance in colonial childrearing.

To some extent, the very lack of historical evidence on childcare suggests the unimportant status of children and mothering. Alice Morse Earle, in 1899 the first historian of childhood in colonial days, considered the "curiously" scant literary sources on her subject a sign that the colonial child was "of as little importance in domestic, social, or ethical relations as his childish successor is of great importance today." She concluded that, in the past, "there was none of that exhaustive study of the motives, thoughts, and actions of a child which is now rife."[54]

What Earle perceived as merely curious Philippe Ariès made a foundation of his theory of childhood. Childhood as we know it, argues Ariès, did not exist in the early modern period but emerged as a distinct phase of life in the sixteenth and seventeenth centuries. Until then, he writes, parents regarded children as little adults. Ariès draws his picture of child life from French society, and other historians who have considered specific aspects of childcare in other European societies find exceptions to his theories. For instance, English and American Puritans thought of children as both innocent and depraved beings; David Stannard suggests that this contradictory view implies that they considered childhood a unique state.[55] But in a general sense Ariès's judgment that the child did not take a central place in the family until recent centuries appears to be accurate.

Every society recognizes its children. The important question is not whether childhood existed before modern times but rather what was different about the way adults treated children. A long view of Anglo-

American family life presents us with significantly different patterns of ideal and actual child life in the seventeenth and twentieth centuries. We value an affectionate relationship between parent and child, and we consider each child a unique individual who deserves to be protected during the child's long years of growth and education. In the seventeenth and early eighteenth centuries children were not protected during privileged years of youth; they began contributing to the subsistence of their families at an early age. Exacting obedience from children mattered more to parents than obtaining their affection, and strong expressions of indifference, hostility, and fear commonly tinged the relationships of parents and child.

When did Americans begin to treat their children in a modern, familiar way? The answer to this, the most elementary of historical inquiries, has as much to do with the history of women as it does with the history of children. At the same time that childrearing became more specialized and sentimentalized in the late eighteenth and early nineteenth centuries, it also became more clearly a feminine task. In other words, when children acquired new importance as individuals, the social role of mothers became more important too. The status of women and that of children are mutually dependent: when Americans began to speculate on the social contribution of women, they also emphasized in a novel way the importance of mothering young children.

These changes in perceptions of children and motherhood roughly coincided with changes in fertility and childbirth practices; for if a new emphasis on childrearing required a more positive view of women, it also required a more positive view of each child as an individual. Such a perception of children was practical only if women had fewer of them, allowing mothers to devote more time and energy to the physical and moral development of each child. The attention that mothers lavished on each child as an individual began at birth—as childbirth came to be seen as an infrequent, private, and potentially dangerous event—and continued throughout childhood and adolescence.

CHAPTER 4

The Occupation of Motherhood: 1750–1850

The new emphasis on motherhood as women's major task in life manifested itself in several ways during the early decades of the nineteenth century. Most obviously, didactic literature on family life expanded enormously and proclaimed more and more strongly women's importance as mothers. Legal changes supported the belief that mothers were the most important influence on their children's development by softening men's exclusive control over their wives and children and by giving women more rights within the family. Most important, the activities of women themselves showed that they adopted wholeheartedly what many were to call their occupation of motherhood.

A special literature on motherhood developed in the nineteenth century, a literature distinguished not only by its subject, childrearing, but by its audience: women. One of the first books on childrearing that we know American women studied was John Locke's *Thoughts Concerning Education.* Written in 1690 and addressed to fathers and tutors, Locke's treatise outlined a plan for rearing English gentlemen from the cradle. When Eliza Pickney read it in 1745, and Martha Ramsay in the 1790s, they had to overlook Locke's warnings that mothers and maids were agents who would subvert a philosopher's designs in the nursery by refusing to feed, bathe, and dress a child according to his plan.[1]

The number of English childrearing manuals written for women increased during the eighteenth century. One that particularly interested Abigail Adams and Mercy Otis Warren, entitled *On the Management and Education of Children*, was written by a man under the pseudonym Juliana Seymour, an indication that although men were still in the business of writing advice to women, at least one of them recognized that women were more likely to accept advice on motherhood from other women.[2] Indigenous American literature on family life proliferated rapidly after 1800, acquiring a prominent place on publishers' lists in the nineteenth century.

The form of the literature varied. American pamphlets printed around 1800 fall into the hallowed genre of reprinted sermons, such as the Congregational minister, Jesse Appleton's, *Discourse Delivered before the Members of the Portsmouth Female Asylum* (Portsmouth, N.H., 1806). Essays that contained advice and treatises on the moral and physical culture of children, hundreds of pages long, also appeared. Sometimes authors of manuals adopted the popular epistolary style, as Seymour did, but as the nineteenth century progressed most authors eschewed the personal, confidential tone of letters and lectured with the full authority of physicians and educators. Early examples of the detached and definitive voice speaks in Dr. William Buchan's much-reprinted manual *Advice to Mothers on the Subject of Their Own Health; and on the Means of Promoting the Health, Strength, and Beauty of Their Offspring* (London, 1803) in *The Mother's Book of Lydia Child* (Boston, 1831), and in William Alcott's treatise *The Young Mother* (Boston, 1836). Periodicals also circulated advice for mothers. Initially articles with what eighteenth-century authors loved to title "Useful Advice to Married Ladies" appeared randomly in American magazines, but soon after 1800 the first of the long-lived "home and health" journals for women appeared, followed by magazines devoted entirely to the subject of childrearing: the *Mother's Magazine*, first published in 1832; *The Mother's Assistant* in 1841; and a *Parents' Magazine* that ran from 1840 to 1850.[3]

Though varied in form and written by men and women of different religious, educational, and medical convictions, a common theme ran through this literature: there is no influence as important in the training of children as that of the mother. At mid-century the Reverend David Strong forcefully stated this fundamental principle of modern family life in the pages of *The Mother's Assistant*. "No one" but the mother, he explained, "can have so intense an interest in the welfare of the child." No one could administer to its wants with so much tenderness. No one could be with the child so much, and be so intimately concerned with its physical, mental, and moral growth. Strong concuded that the nature of temporal and eternal life of "any generation" depended entirely on the quality of maternal care. Childrearing was an awesome maternal responsibility.[4]

There are, of course, limits to the conclusions that we can derive from surveying literature such as Strong's essay on "maternal responsibility," which at times historians have failed to recognize. Academics, educators, and historians have more than an ordinary fondness for the printed word and have, despite evidence to the contrary, faith in its efficacy. Accordingly, some of the first historians who wrote about women and the family tended to analyze literature as if it explained life.[5] As some scholars are now reminding us about fiction and didactic literature, what ought to have been is not always what was. There is not necessarily a causal relationship between official advice and actual practice. We cannot assume that parents learned childrearing from manuals or that they treated their children differently merely because advisors told them to do so. Neither can we assume that the advice in manuals reflects a universal opinion to which Americans were uniformly exposed in the nineteenth century. The literature has an unquestionable bias toward educated, middle-class, native-born American readers and writers.[6]

Despite these limitations, childrearing literature offers some important insights into women's changing role as mothers. To begin with, we cannot dismiss all didactic literature as an expression of the ideal, alien to the experience of women. Many of the authors of childcare manuals, some of them women, include case histories and descriptions of their own experiences. Certainly we can use the literature to trace the early intellectual history of assumptions about a mother's role in childcare that later influenced social welfare legislation. The proliferation of literature on childcare also indicates that for one reason or another Americans began to pay for the knowledge of experts on childcare. Significantly, the literature was addressed to mothers, informing us that women confronted new ideals of childrearing; some of them translated advice into practice, occasionally with frustrating consequences. Both authors and audience scrutinized nurseries with a new intensity, and what they saw were impressionable infants in the arms of powerful mothers.

"The truth is daily coming before the public," wrote John Abbott in 1833, "that the influence which is so exerted upon the mind during the first eight or ten years of existence, in a great degree guides the destinies of that mind for time and eternity." Because mothers guarded and guided children during the early years of life, they were, Abbott avowed, "the most powerful influence in the formation of the character of man." Abbott described mother's work as "secret and silent . . . powerful and extensive."[7] Other authors used metaphors, employing the images of a queen or a gardener to convey the nature of maternal influence. A mother was like a gardener, Daniel Chaplin told the Female Society of Groton, Connecticut, in 1814. She had care of plants "naturally crushed and ill-shapen," which with her attention and with the blessing of God "must be made straight by culture."[8] Margaret Coxe, writing a few decades later during Victoria's reign, thought that the immense power mothers wielded over their children and society could best be understood as a species of royal might. Each American mother, whatever her position in society, "as a moral guardian, will be placed on the same footing with the youthful sovereign of the British empire."[9] As another Victorian said it, "The hand that rocks the cradle, is the hand that rules the world."[10]

Like the province controlled by another would-be emperor, the area of a mother's rule fell into three parts—at least, the counselors of childrearing subdivided maternal responsibility into physical, mental, and moral categories.[11]

Departing from older conventions, the literature advised mothers to take complete physical care of their children and to treat them according to the laws of health. Repeatedly, authorities asserted that no prudent mother would give her infant to a mercenary nurse. "Trust not your treasure too much to hirelings, have it under your superintendence, both night and day," said Mrs. Lydia Sigourney who, like other counselors, considered it dangerous to "put children out of the way

with nurses."[12] The advice givers meant "nurse" in its most fundamental sense. They encouraged all mothers to breast-feed their infants
and proposed also that women release children from swaddling bands
and provide them with fresh air and frequent exercise. Given such attention, more infants would survive the first years of life.

The physician who in 1844 appended a supplementary chapter to
the first American edition of Louisa Barwell's *Infant Treatment* confronted infant mortality statistics very similar to those Benjamin Franklin
had observed a century earlier. Between 1832 and 1842, the years for
which he examined the death registers of major American cities, about
one-half of all the children born still died of disease before their fifth
birthday. But in the 1840s, these deaths seemed outrageous, not "part
of the established order of nature, or of the systematic arrangements
of Divine Providence," but the result of human stupidity and neglect.
Americans had been justly accused of undervaluing human life, wrote
this anonymous physician, and the proof was "not in the frequency of
duels, of savage personal combats, lynch law, the bursting of steam-
boat boilers, or the destruction of rail-road cares." It lay rather in the
general, "and we fear wilful ignorance of the laws of life."[13] Those
laws were accessible to every thinking mother and nurse between the
covers of his annotated edition of *Infant Treatment* and other books.

Though many other Americans living in the 1840s shared this New
York physician's confidence that much disease could be prevented
through healthful diet and dress, it is incorrect to describe the plen-
tiful advice on children's health only as one enthusiasm of antebellum
health reformers.[14] British and American physicians advocated changing methods of infant care long before Catharine Beecher or Mary Gove
Nichols lectured on the subject. English literature, including Dr. William Cadogan's pioneer *Essay Upon Nursing and Management of Children*,
had circulated in America after the 1770s, and by 1800 American authors contributed similar insights on feeding and dressing small children. Although the overall mortality rate for infants had not changed
greatly between 1740 and 1840 (and perhaps even increased after
dropping about 1800), the recommended methods of infant care had.

After 1750 physicians endeavored to persuade women that the only
healthy thing to put in an infant's mouth was its mother's breast. Wet-
nursing by careless or sick nurses and early day feeding deprived ba-

bies of nutrition and affection, they charged, and really amounted to infanticide. Indeed, Cadogan remarked caustically that the ancient custom of exposing babies to wild beasts or drowning them "would certainly be a much quicker and more humane way of dispatching them."[15]

Doctors described how mothers and nurses began poisoning children within minutes after they emerged from the womb. Instead of letting an infant draw the first scanty fluid from its mother's breasts, women immediately gave it to a nurse with flowing milk, crammed it with other food "as if it had come into the world famished," or dosed it with purgatives or laudanum. A dab of butter with sugar, a little softened bread and roast pork, a mixture of soot and water, toddy, and catnip tea with a drop of gin in it were among the substances doctors repeatedly saw fed to newborns.[16] If an infant survived this banquet, nurses supplemented breast milk with pap and panada, bread slightly boiled in milk, water, or beer, and gave it biscuits and meat before it had teeth to chew. Doctors estimated that infants who were "dry fed" pap and cow's milk sucked from a sponge or rag stuck in a bottle had the least chance of living. Although ignorant of microorganisms, they knew that the sour milk of cows fed city slops was deadly to children. It did not surprise doctors that intestinal diseases were the greatest cause of child death.[17]

The doctors who first analyzed infant feeding, and the lay health reformers who lectured and wrote on the subject later in the nineteenth century, maintained that most of the fatal infantile diarrheas would disappear if babies consumed a diet of mother's milk. This, they suggested, should be offered at regular feedings for at least eight and perhaps as long as fourteen months. Mothers should introduce children to solid food slowly, never give them bread, meat, and cake before the teeth appeared, and cease administering opiate "cordial" and "soothing syrups" to fussy babies.[18] On this regime mothers as well as their offspring would flourish. Spared milk fever, nursing mothers would enjoy a clear complexion; a good appetite; cheerful spirits; and, one New York midwife wrote, a respite from pregnancy.[19]

Writers stressed the emotional benefits of breast-feeding almost as much as the physical ones, asserting that a paid nurse gave mere nourishment; a mother provided watchful tenderness as well. While nursing, she began to observe her child's character and transmitted her "agreeable impressions" and sympathies to it. Naturally, mothers cherished the children they nursed more than those suckled by wet nurses. Midwife Mary Watkins described nursing as "a very high source of pleasure" for a woman, "which also remarkably strengthens her attachment to the infant of her bosom." How much better to encourage this love than to have a stranger alienate mother and child.[20]

Several men, writing in the freer language of the eighteenth century, reassured women that they would also secure their husbands' love by nursing their babies. According to popular wisdom, carnal relations spoiled the milk of nursing mothers. Understandably, some husbands resented the consequent prohibition on marital relations. Parental rather than sexual affection colored the new picture of domestic harmony that they drew. "Believe it not, when it is insinuated that your bosoms are less charming, for having a dear little cherub at your breast," wrote Dr. Hugh Smith. A husband's love could only be aroused by the sight of his nursing wife, "carefully intent upon the preservation of his own image!"[21] Less sentimentally, Dr. Cadogan pointed out that a well-fed child would always be in good humor, so "There would be no fear of offending the husband's ears with the noise of a squalling brat." But, in his opinion, "a man of sense cannot have a prettier rattle (for rattles he must have of one kind or another) than such a young child."[22]

After 1750 the advice literature increasingly told mothers to demonstrate concern for their children by feeding them carefully. For the first time, authorities claimed that the survival and, more interestingly, the happiness of child and parents depended on the strength of the maternal bond. Manuals began to offer detailed instructions on the mechanics of nurture; schedules for first feedings of solid foods; prohibitions on alcohol, bread, coffee, and sweets. No standard feeding schedule emerged in the literature by 1860; here one man advises nursing an infant every three hours; there another says four times within twenty-four hours; and occasionally the advice is to let the child establish its own routine. But, no matter how each prescription differed, the underlying principle was identical. Feeding a child properly required observation, calculation, and concerned attention.

The same values emerged in other advice on the physical care of children. As in their discussions of feeding, advisors pronounced swaddling detrimental to the happiness as well as to the health of children. Their injunctions to unwrap babies from confining clothing, to let them exercise and play, promised more freedom to children—and, as anyone who has ever watched a crawling child knows—demanded more supervision from adults.

In 1809, midwife Watkins begged the women of New York City to study their babies in the evening while they were "taking off its day clothes and swathing it again" for the night. During this interval, usually the only time during the day when an infant's diapers were changed, the child's instinct to be free would be obvious. To support her own observations, Watkins cited Dr. Cadogan, who sixty years before, in his argument against swaddling, had written of "that particular happiness, which a child shows by all its powers of expression, when it is newly undressed. How pleased! How delightful! it is with this new liberty."[23] Nature intended children to be "in perpetual motion," as Watkins put it. Loose flannel gowns and petticoats, tied or taped, were therefore the appropriate garments for babies. Such light clothes would safely cover them (the straight pins used to secure swaddling clothes occasionally penetrated children's bodies) while allowing free motion and additionally making it easier to wash babies "free from stinks and soreness" every day.[24]

Binding American babies tightly in some way was apparently still common in the 1830s, when critics of the practice multiplied. Health reformers and educators joined the physicians who had continued to pronounce swaddling as "decidedly unreasonable, injurious, and cruel."[25] Lecturers such as Mary Gove incorporated denunciations of children's dress and diet into their general crusades to improve the physical health of Americans. Like women's corsets, another object of criticism, infants' garb obstructed circulation, crushed bones, and inhibited breathing. Reformers thought that acquiring an elementary knowledge of human anatomy would stimulate women to loosen children's clothes as well as their own corset laces.[26]

What emerges, then, in didactic literature by the middle of the nineteenth century are recommendations that women assume, as much as possible, complete physical care of their children. A good mother, who understood the rules of health, would spend more time feeding, bathing, and supervising her child, and the words of experts provided indispensable instructions on the mechanics of these tasks. It was a mother's duty to get a treatise on anatomy or childcare, advisors wrote self-consciously, as they recommended the books of Dr. Dewees of Philadelphia, or Catherine Beecher's *Treatise on Domestic Economy*, or Dr. Combe's *Physiology of Digestion*.[27]

Of course, women always had the primary responsiblity for child nurture. What was new was the insistence that women nurture their own children following scientific or "naturally" correct methods. Perhaps more thoroughly innovative were the arguments that mothers rather than fathers should begin to train children's conscience and intellect.

The men and women who taught in New England classrooms had to secure licenses from school boards, but, we read in advice literature, every woman who gave birth automatically acquired a teaching certificate. Writing in 1838, Lydia Sigourney congratulated her readers, who as mothers had advanced to the head of the teaching profession. No superintendent of education could terminate their careers, said Mrs. Sigourney. "You hold that license which authorizes you to teach always. You have attained that degree in the College of Instruction, by which your pupils are in your presence continually."[28]

The literature generally accredited this degree explaining that mothers possessed superior talents as pedagogues. Because they had the advantage of daily association with children, mothers would scale lessons to suit the capacity of each child. Furthermore, women inherently had two qualities desirable in a teacher of the young, patience and love. This line of reasoning proved so compelling that it also came to constitute one important justification for training women to be paid primary school teachers.[29]

Heretofore, a teacher's most valuable asset had been the strength of his whipping arm. As Anne Kuhn points out in her study of the mother's role in childhood education, when nineteenth-century educators associated the teaching of the young with maternal nature, they rejected the old system of forcing precocious mental discipline. Adopting a more liberal attitude toward child growth, they condemned parents and teachers who trained three- and four-year-olds to read by memorizing long exercises and who kept seven-year-olds sitting motionless for hours on school benches under threat of beating.[30] How much better, they thought, if the young child's intellect developed gradually in domestic surroundings, under the sympathetic tutelage of a mother.

Long before teaching the child to read and write, she would encourage its infantile powers of reasoning by turning daily activities, such as playing in the parlor, into lessons. The manuals showed how a mother could do this by letting her child explore its environment, by giving it information and making it draw associations. Almira Phelps, who had taught at her sister Emma Willard's seminary in Troy, New York, published her journal of the first year of her baby's life, which offered American mothers a case history of infant education. Phelps claimed to have developed her boy's curiosity and perception by letting him shake a box of colored wafers until it popped open. When hundreds of bright, round pieces fell about him, she knew that he had conquered a difficulty and had made a discovery. "No botanist on finding a new plant, mineralogist at the sight of a new specimen, or mathematician on the solution of a difficult problem could feel greater pleasure than was now apparent in this little miniature man at the sight of the broke box and scattered wafers."[31] After writing that it was not enough to play pat-a-cake with babies, Lydia Child supplied models of superior mother-child exchanges. "This ball is *round*. This little table is *square*. Now George knows what *round* and *square* mean," reads an example similar to many others in advice literature.[32]

Thus, taking advantage of her child's growing curiosity, a mother could teach it colors and shapes by comparing objects in the house and garden; then she could show it how to count its fingers and the buttons on jackets. When a child reached the age of three, it would be capable of retaining more abstract information recited to it, such as the Lord's Prayer.[33] However, at this stage, as well as later when she taught her child to read and write, the lessons should not degenerate into mere tests of a child's memory of the names of kings, towns, rivers, and dates of battles and treaties. *The Mother's Friend* termed these mnemonic exercises, beloved of grammar school teachers, unmerciful loads on young minds. Good daily lessons should be short, frequent, and taught by conversing in a series of questions and answers.[34]

Amazingly, no one appears to have dignified this style of teaching by calling it the Socratic method. In their effort to convince mothers, if not also themselves, of the gravity of teaching two-year-olds the difference between round and square, educators described the process of childrearing in sophisticated terms. Jacob Abbott titled children's first attempts to learn colors and shapes "Philosophy," because in them children worked to discover the nature of things.[35] "Optics is a favorite study of little children," Almira Phelps wrote, explaining her son's fascination with mirrors; and his persistent brushes against a hot stove were "experiments upon the capacity of metals for caloric."[36] Such evaluation of childish activity reinforced the educator's message that every early encounter with the world irrevocably molded a child's life. No sensation, no idea, was irrelevant to a baby. "Every mother ought to know," Almira Phelps warned, "that as soon as her child can distinguish her from strangers it is capable of receiving impressions which may prove favorable or unfavorable to its future well-being, affecting its moral and religious character."[37] If moral faculties unfolded in infancy along with intellectual talents, as the educators and ministers who wrote advice literature assumed, then a Christian mother's task was of supreme importance. She had to begin moral education of her children when they were babes in arms, or their souls—and society—would suffer.[38]

As we have seen, Protestant ministers and educators had always emphasized the necessity for parents to give children early religious training. However, in the late eighteenth century, they began to characterize this education differently. While continuing to maintain that obedience to divine and parental authority was the first lesson that a child ought to learn, they described the process of religious education as one of instilling right values and encouraging a child's natural instincts to do good, rather than one of beating deviltry out of it. At the same time, educators transferred the primary responsibility for religious and ethical training of children to mothers.

Ministers conceded that the religious education of children depended "principally" on the mother. She, the Reverend Joseph Lathrop told the women of Springfield's Female Association, knew her children better than did anyone else.[39] She alone could "improve the numberless occasions which open the mind for instruction," said Jacob Abbott. Almost 200 years after Anne Hutchinson was banished from Massachusetts for holding prayer meetings in her house, Abbott concluded that "The quiet fireside is the most sacred sanctuary; maternal affection is the most eloquent pleader, and an obedient child is the most promising subject of religious impression."[40]

Fathers appeared as peripheral figures in domestic sanctuaries. "Early Religious Impressions the Appropriate Business of Mothers" reads the title of an essay that appeared in the *Mother's Magazine*, an accurate summary of the overwhelming direction of thought on religious education. Catechisms and instructive dialogues featured mothers in the interrogative role, and essays on education reminded mothers that it was *their* privilege to lead children "at the first dawn of intelligence" to the "babe of Bethlehem and the man of Calvary."[41] Occasionally someone granted that fathers also influenced their children's moral development, though mainly by marrying a virtuous woman. A man's "first duty" toward the religious education of his children was to be "most scrupulous" in the selection of a wife. Since he "cannot know much of his children in their earlier years," he ought to be quite certain that their mother would surround them with pious attention. By the time a father could counsel them in adulthood, the damage of her failings would be irreversible. Though a man might hire instructors for his children, George Burnap warned, if their mother were negligent toward their studies, his money would be thrown away. In vain would a father struggle to keep them out of bad company, if their mother suffered them to go where they pleased. Burnap, for one, abdicated the responsibility for moral education, leaving it entirely to mothers.[42]

Ideally, a mother began her child's moral education by giving catechism lessons in articles of faith and in scripture and by teaching it how to pray. To equate high moral training with the scrupulous practice of religious rituals (in the case of advice literature, specifically Protestant practice) is to define morality in perhaps its narrowest sense, but the ministers and secular moralists who wrote didactic literature had little doubt that an outwardly professing Christian was likely to be morally upright. They emphasized the importance of early training, stressing that morals degenerated in families that failed to pray. It was maintained that even a child of age one could comprehend the meaning of family prayer at table, that a two-year-old could be moved by the sight of its praying mother, and that a three-year-old could observe the Sabbath in a churchgoing family.[43]

Mothers were therefore advised to begin teaching toddlers "daily self-examination" and to instruct them to hallow the Sabbath and donate their pennies to benevolent societies. At the first "signs of sin" in a child, a Christian mother should "quietly" lead it away to obtain help from above. "Without a word of reproof," advised "B.," a contributor to the *Mother's Magazine*, she should simply say, "My child, you need a helper; you are in danger and are weak; sin is strong, Satan is strong, but God is able to subdue both."[44] While "B." conceived of religious education as a process of rescue, other writers suggested that mothers act before intransigence manifested itself and that they instill the habit of prayer by beginning Bible lessons every morning when children turned two.[45]

Protestants linked this specifically religious education with broad American goals of social progress. Lessons in scripture and prayer would develop children's conscience and benevolent feelings, they asserted, and thereby produce good citizens as well as good Christians. Repeatedly we read in the literature of the ninetenth century that the character of public life depends in great measure on the quality of the moral instruction mothers give to their children. An early expression of this, an almost universal assumption among the educated in nineteenth-century America, appears in a sermon of the Reverend William Lyman's, who declared in 1802 that the basis of public virtue, union, peace, and happiness in society "depended on the way women molded the moral sentiments of children. Mothers do, in a sense, hold the reigns of government and sway the ensigns of national prosperity and glory," he told his New London listeners, assuring them that maternal influence would "drive discord, infidelity and licentiousness from our land."[46] However, the health of the federal Union still appeared precarious in 1851, when the Reverend William Thayer called American mothers to give their nation the citizens it desperately needed, the "public men of master minds and tried religious principles," "the citizens of enlarged benevolence," the "faithful and fearless ministers of the Gospel." "Hear then, ye Mothers," he cried, asking the by then rhetorical question, "Who but ye can form the character of rising generations to be Reformers?"[47]

Occasionally advisors specified public problems, other than general moral breakdown, that mothers could cure by proper instruction. The national mania for money-getting was one, said Sarah Hale, the editor of the *Ladies' Magazine* in 1830; she believed that in their pursuit of the almighty dollar Americans had elevated avarice and self-love into virtues. Americans could shake off selfishness only if mothers began to teach their children that money is worthless unless it is used to do good. They could do this by refusing to hire children to peform tasks of any kind and by substituting the motto "Time is the opportunity for doing good" for "that heartless maxim 'Time is money.' " Beyond this, suggested the enterprising editor Hale, donating pennies to pay for the completion of the Bunker Hill Monument would give the children of America a splendid lesson in love of country and the pleasures of doing good.[48]

However ingenious Sarah Hale's plans for forming benevolent citizens were, in the nineteenth century the epitome of maternal influence on public morals was represented by the relationship between Mary Ball Washington and her son George. Myths about the mother of Washington commanded a preeminent place among the many stories about the "mothers of great men" first published during the century. Mary Washington had worthy companions in the pantheon of popular sentiment. There were the ancients Cornelia, mother of the Gracchi, who displayed her sons to her wealthy friends saying, "These are my jewels"; and Monica, whose son, the "poet and preacher" Augustine, acknowledged her influence in his *Confessions*. Among the moderns stood the mother of Napoleon, whose son "declared frequently his debt to his mother"; the mothers of Kant and Hegel, who had led their sons' thoughts into "vast fields of speculation"; and, after the American Civil War, the mothers of Abraham Lincoln and Thaddeus Stevens.[49] But, as the subject of at least two full-scale biographies and numerous short morality tales, the mother of America's first president attracted the most admiration.

A common moral illuminated all the maternal morality stories: a great man is the product of his early childhood upbringing, and therefore all his public actions are explicable by the kind of care that his mother gave him. Lord Byron's mother, the stories alleged, taunted him about his deformities, taught him to defy authority and indulge in sin, and "made her son a curse to his fellow men." Benedict Arnold's mother allowed the future traitor to "destroy insects, to mutilate toads, to steal the eggs of the humming bird, and torture quiet domestic animals."[50]

George Washington's mother, however, was made of better stuff. She taught her boy obedience, moral courage, and virtue. Had she been a careless, indulgent parent, ran the stories, "The unchecked energies of Washington might have elevated him to the throne of a tyrant."[51]

Imaginative moralists described many occasions when Mary Washington curbed the will and stimulated the conscience of her son. To the biography of Washington they added the story of the sorrel colt, a twin of the cherry tree story, in which George's mother, asks the uncomfortable question, "Who has seen my fine sorrel colt?"[52] Then there was the story, also often printed in schoolbooks, of the teenage George's renunciation of a naval career at his mother's request. "Order your trunk ashore, and return your uniform, my son, if you do not wish to crush your mother's heart," declaimed Mrs. Washington in one bit of fanciful dialogue.[53] The one story probably closest to fact was the marquis de Lafayette's visit to Mrs. Washington in 1784, when in response to his praise of her son, she replied, "I am not surprised at what George has done, for he was always a good boy."[54] Lafayette is suposed to have returned to Mount Vernon certain that he had identified the source of Washington's greatness, saying, "I have seen the only Roman matron living at this day." But the only thing we can be sure of is that the people who told the story in the nineteenth century thought that *they* had identified the source of Washington's greatness.[55]

The unhappy truth is that George Washington maintained a filial but firmly distant relationship with his mother, by reliable accounts an overbearing, miserly woman who in her old age embarrassed the president by falsely claiming that she was starving because he refused to support her. As a youth Washington had escaped to the household of his brother Lawrence, and in manhood he visited the home of his sister rather than stay with his mother.[56] People in the nineteenth century created the morally thrilling, if fictitious, stories. Their faith in the supreme importance of mothering led them to claim that the mother of Washington deserved the nation's reverence and gratitude.

Another species of stories underscored the moral power of mothers by providing proof that if, despite her efforts, a child proved wayward, a mother could still save him with prayer. Sometimes maternal prayer miraculously rescued a good child from danger, as in the story of the sailor who survived a fall from the topmast to the deck and told his astonished captain, "This is the hour when my mother prays for me, and I could not be hurt while she was praying."[57] More frequently, a mother's prayer restored a wanderer to the path of virtue, if not also to her arms. As mentioned earlier, the modern prodigal returned to a maternal, rather than a paternal, embrace. Apparently an unregenerate lot, the men of the American merchant marine frequently figured in these rescue stories. They succumbed, sobbing, at the doors of seamen's missions, when preachers asked, "Suppose your mother were here now, what advice would she give you?" And they crawled home to die, so disfigured by dissipation that only their forgiving mothers could recognize them.[58] And the mere thought of their praying mothers also prevented politicians and businessmen from evildoing. Such was the experience of "a distinguished public man of Indiana," who did not abscond down the Mississippi with the $22,000 that he had been entrusted to deliver to Cincinnati. He saw the image of his aged mother, sitting on a bench in a humble farmhouse "reading to her boy from the Oracles of God," and went to Cincinnati instead of to New Orleans.[59]

We do not have to search hard for the meanings of these miracle stories because the authors were unable to resist hitting their readers with the blunt end of a moral. Two lessons generally struck the reader's eyes. One, inescapable in the prodigal son stories, was that the childhood lessons and prayers of a mother stayed with her children forever. "A *good* mother *never dies*," wrote one author as he introduced the story of J——, another of the legion of dissipated and skeptical men rescued by maternal prayer.[60] As long as a mother could pray, and as long as a child could remember its praying mother, moralists claimed, virtue existed in its life.

The other common lesson was that powerful love motivated mothers' concern for their children. To use the epigram of another moralist, "The heart of a mother can never grow cold." Nothing children could do would alienate a mother's love. They might move to the other side of the globe and live like infidels, but God had planted a deep, unquenchable, irrepressible love for her offspring in their mother's heart. From the moment that a woman first gazed on her newborn to the instant she died, she never remitted her care for her child. Compared with her love, the love of a father, of brothers and sisters, seemed to be secondary, "the result of habit and association."[61]

This statement—which dismisses paternal feeling as the product of mere habit—and the magazine for mothers in which it appeared in 1839 are historically remarkable. They are manifestations of ideas that developed among the educated late in the eighteenth century (and certainly late in the history of Western thought). The argument that the care of young children is an exacting, time-consuming, and important activity that should be the center of women's lives had emerged clearly in didactic literature by 1830, along with the innovative contention that the mother is socially the most important parent.

By the middle of the nineteenth century, the expert had also assumed a role in childrearing, even if only by implication; the literature inherently boosted the importance of the ministers and educators who wrote it. The historical beginnings of the trend to rely on the advice of experts in childcare emerged most clearly in the treatises written by physicians on the physical care of babies, though their so-called scientific expertise did not dominate childrearing advice until the late nineteenth century.

We can consider the proliferation of advice literature and stories in the nineteenth century as a symptom of intense interest in childrearing, and perhaps also as an attempt to justify it. A more difficult question is *why* Americans revised their definitions of the mother's role in childrearing when they did. The timing suggests that revision of the maternal role complemented and even facilitated the changes of modernization.

It is a well-known fact that the material processes of modernization—urbanization and industrialization—accelerated early in the nineteenth century. And at the same time, the thoughtful recognized that these material changes affected families. However, the familiarity of the explanations should not diminish our appreciation of the fact that the economic reorganization of America substantially altered family life.

Modernization did not transform America at a uniform pace; for example, older work habits and family organization persisted among ethnically distinct immigrant groups, even in the highly industrialized cities of the early twentieth century.[62] Yet we can discern a well-established, characteristically modern urban and economic order before the Civil War. The changes appeared in their earliest and most pronounced forms in the Northeast—the location of an economically and culturally linked urban network and also the home of a substantial number of well-educated, commercially oriented middle-class people who, not coincidentally, were the first to write and read the literature on childrearing.

Like the cathedral, which had become a visible symbol of the Middle Ages, the factory has become a visible symbol of the modern world; these are the buildings where people congregated to perform the rituals of most meaning to their society. The metaphor may be attractive because it leads to striking and disturbing comparisons between spires and smokestacks, saints and steam engines; but it is also misleading because it confuses modernization with industrialization. The cities and commerce of western Europe and America, and the ambitions of entrepreneurs, began taking modern form before many factories were built.

In America cities began to assume a modern aspect in the middle of the eighteenth century. The large seaport cities had always been the administrative centers of the colonies, but their population increased and their commercial function was exaggerated in the decades before the Revolution. In Boston, Philadelphia, and New York a growing class of merchants hinged their fortunes on the uncertainties of coastal, Caribbean, and transatlantic trade; the number of clerks, agents, marine-insurance brokers, bankers, and lawyers multiplied and watched the fluctuations of trade with as much anxiety as did the merchants themselves. By enlarging their parochial horzons, global commerce made businessmen cosmopolitan as well as wealthy. Citizen entrepreneurs voluntarily created libraries, fire companies, and street improvement societies to enhance the cities that were the homes of their ventures.[63]

Imperial trade restrictions and revenue laws, the depressions of the 1760s, the crisis of the Revolutionary War, and the uncertainties of confederation disrupted commerce for twenty years; but ultimately the Revolution encouraged the American economy to move again in the direction that it had started to take before 1760. With political independence and a federal constitution, Americans institutionalized nationalism and increased their incentive to cultivate interstate and international markets as well as domestic manufacturing. The *Report on Manufactures* commissioned by Congress from Secretary of the Treasury Alexander Hamilton in 1791, which enthusiastically supported the efforts of manufacturing societies to set up textile factories in almost every state, identified a national goal of industrial development, though it announced the birth of the textile industry prematurely. Almost all the industrial enterprises of the 1790s died quickly, as did most of the factories founded during the embargo of 1808. Employing relatively few laborers and producing modest amounts of cloth, American factories were economically insignificant until the 1820s. Primarily, they demonstrated the presence of an industrial consciousness.[64]

Yet during the same years of the abortive attempts to establish textile factories, the American economy modernized in other significant ways. Economic and urban historians have catalogued the transformations that occurred between 1760 and 1820. Taking the state of Massachusetts, Richard Brown describes the emergence of an urban network united by efficient systems of communication. In this state, people moved from farms to Boston and to middle-sized towns of 1,000 to 2,000 population well before large-scale industrial development commenced. At least 20 percent of these town dwellers engaged in nonagricultural callings that permitted some leisure and connected them, by post, with towns throughout the Northeast. These people valued the multiple opportunities provided by towns, rather than any single local or familial authority, and demonstrated their concern for improving themselves and their environment by founding nearly 2,000 voluntary associations. Though the Massachusetts landscape appeared almost as pastoral in 1800 as it had in 1760, its thriving towns were filled with men and women of broadened outlook and ambitions, some of whom were accumulating, through mercantile enterprises, the capital that would construct the mills of Lowell and Waltham.[65]

Urban society, with its modern approaches to time and trade, extended into rural America at the outset of the nineteenth century, though the fundamental division of labor between commercial central places and the agricultural hinterlands was little disturbed until about 1815. After that time, the rate of urban population growth and the contours of city borders changed dramatically. At varying but highly accelerated paces, the cities of the New England and central Atlantic states absorbed hundreds of thousands of immigrants and appropriated miles of new territory. Indeed, urbanization in the Northeast, when measured in rate of growth rather than in sheer numbers, peaked before the Civil War.[66] The largest cities gained population but remained commercially oriented; factories and industrial laborers concentrated in newer satellite cities, which had cheaper land and frequently rivers to power machinery.[67]

The growth of manufacturing satellites and residential suburbs was a remarkable feature of American urban development well before mid-century. It is important to recognize not only that the population of New York City leaped from 124,000 inhabitants in 1820 to 516,000 in 1850 but also that more people who worked in the commercial core of the city lived a short distance away in the suburbs. Large residential suburbs surrounded Boston, Philadelphia, and New York in the 1850s, a fact that has been obscured because cities later annexed these areas, transforming them into neighborhoods. New York City, for example, expanded its area from 2 to 129 square miles in 1854, boosting its population by thousands, by incorporating independent suburbs into its boundaries.[68]

By the time of the Civil War, then, several million Americans lived in the large cities of the Northeast, and many more lived in towns connected commercially and culturally with the big cities. Even western migration in the nineteenth century was characteristically modern, commercial, and tightly tied to the East. All this means that a substantial number of men and women had separated themselves directly from agricultural labor. The rhythms of family life that accompany subsistence farming changed in cities, where men worked in central business districts and women in the residences beyond.

During the decades from 1820 to 1860, industrial manufacturing and technology also had entered the lives of most Americans decisively, especially in the Northeast. A truly national exchange of regionally specialized agricultural and manufactured products existed by 1860. Americans created a national market, in which farmers grew single cash crops for market rather than for home use. Subsistence farming and domestic manufacturing became unattractive and unnecessary. Canals and, later, railroads and shallow-draft steamboats as well as coastal vessels continuously carried the products of New England factories to the South and Northwest, returning with wheat and corn from western farms and mills and cotton from southern fields. In forty years America had become an industrial nation second only to Britain in manufacturing, and domestic rather than foreign buyers purchased most American-made products.[69]

Observant Americans living in the cities and towns of the Northeast and Midwest recognized early that the commercial production and distribution of commodities had relieved women of household manufacture. Indeed, some people believed that the question of women's right to a political or professional life—which was pushed into the newspapers by the Women's Rights Convention at Seneca Falls, New York, in 1848—was a consequence of this revolution in the American economy. When all manufactures were domestic, Theodore Parker told an audience in the Boston Music Hall, then domestic work consumed all the time of "able-headed" women. But in 1853, "the flour mills of Rochester and Boston take the place of the pestle and mortar and the hand-mill of the Old Testament, [and] Lowell and Lawrence are two enormous Old-Testament women, spinning and weaving year out and year in, day and night both." When butchers, bakers, tailors, cooks, and gasmakers added their contributions to households, the women of Boston had time for other things.[70]

The statistics available on home manufacturing support Parker's impressions. In most parts of the country, household manufacture, other than food preparation, had largely disappeared by 1860, declining first in the East and persisting longer in the Midwest and in some southern states, where transportation was more difficult or expensive. The speed with which the women of New England abandoned the burden of domestic textile production astonished the secretary of the treasury in 1833, who reported that during the six previous years household manufactures of cloth had dropped between 50 and 90 percent. The later figures for New York State allow us to measure each woman's freedom from the loom by inches of fabric; in New York per capita yardage produced in homes declined from 8.95 in 1825 to barely .27 in 1855, and the women in counties most remote from the Erie Canal did most of the weaving.[71] Because American factories were so productive and transportation was so swift and regular, the system of home manufacture did not move west after 1840; the women who settled the plains and the Far West purchased their cloth and household goods.[72]

Manufacturers had taken spinning, weaving, and later sewing outside women's homes. Women could buy blankets, rugs, and stockings; they could purchase yards of coarser cotton fabric for table linen, sheets, towels, and clothing instead of twisting and weaving the threads themselves. In household account books, we can read the notations that reveal housewives' increasing reliance on manufactured basic commodities as well as luxury goods. Between 1821 and 1824 Hannah Hickok Smith, a prosperous farm matron in a commercial Connecticut town, purchased foodstuffs that had formerly been luxuries (raisins, sugar, wine, coffee, tea); construction materials (pine boards and nails); household items (soap, teacups, tinwear, pins); and at least eleven different kinds of fabric, four kinds of yarn and thread, leather and buttons, shawls, bonnets, dresses, stockings, and kid gloves. She also paid for a dressmaker with money earned from the sale of the farm's grain and animals.[73]

The development of a market economy and industrial manufacture did not, of course, mean that all or even most American women suddenly had time to be idle or develop talents other than domestic ones. Some farm women followed the spindle and loom into the factories; until the mid-1840s, the overwhelming number of workers tending machinery in textile factories were unmarried young women. Other northeastern women formed the links holding together the chain of the "putting-out" system of manufacture that flourished from 1840 to 1860. In their homes, they stitched together the machine-made components of stockings and shoes.[74] However, the norm for the married adult woman (and the low wages and temporary nature of women's job reflected this well into the twentieth century) remained unpaid household work.

However, the character of work connected with the house changed, especially for middle-class women. The labor of purchase replaced that of production during the course of the nineteenth century as urban women devoted more time to household shopping. To people who, in 1900, witnessed the crowds of female shoppers in the business district of American cities, the trip downtown and the wanderings from counter to counter fingering and pricing seemed to be the chief employment of tens of thousands of American women.[75] Women also became more preoccupied with keeping their houses, clothing, and persons clean; it was the nineteenth-century urban housewife who made cleanliness a common virtue.[76] But childrearing appears to have expanded into the most time-consuming of domestic activities, the one that well-to-do urban women like Mary Lee of Boston began to call their "occupation" early in the nineteenth century. In letters to husband and friends, Lee, like other women of her class, detailed the moods and accomplishments of her babies, admitted to feeling an awesome responsibility to rear them properly, and also confessed that taking care of children gave her something useful to do. "I so much desire to feel as if I was of consequence to someone," she wrote to her husband in 1813, "that if the child has the finger ache, or nurse looks pale, I immediately think I cannot possibly leave them and thus gain my point."[77]

At the time that Mary Lee wrote this insight, her husband was trading in Calcutta, a separation that emphasized to her the importance of her parental role. For other women, a husband's daily migration to office or business downtown could serve the same purpose. By mid-century the most respectable addresses in large cities no longer were located as close as possible to the center of town as the geography of American cities began assuming the characteristically modern separation of residential and working districts. Merchants and manufacturers, lawyers and physicians took their homes away from the noise and smell of commerce, a move clear in eastern cities by the 1840s, and discernible even in the newer cities of Chicago and San Francisco by 1860.[78] Professionals and businessmen divided their families from their offices with a long walk or a horsecar or ferry ride and thus disassociated themselves from the daily lives of their small children.

The Americans who wrote about childrearing recognized that the division between home and father's workplace had helped to inaugurate a change in women's work role by exaggerating the maternal responsibility in childrearing. They also thought that the vigor with which American men pursued their work further distracted paternal attention from families. American fathers—some dared to say the mechanics and the farmers as well as the professionals—exerted themselves not merely to support their families but to increase their wealth. They gave their whole time to "the labors of the study and public duties," or they returned home from the counting room or the shop "fatigued with the cares of business." These men either could not or did not want to spend the evenings and Sundays with their families, arbitrating domestic controversies. They abhorred "being saluted with complaints, how bad the children had behaved, by their mother, or clamors for sugar plums or rocking horses from the discontented urchins."[79]

Admitting this situation to be a fact of life, most authors of didactic literature in the early nineteenth century briskly proceeded to outline the enlarged responsibilities of mothers. They did not, on the whole, dwell on the unfortunate fate of children deprived of paternal attention. The "abnormal fatherless children of the suburbs," or of the poor, became the objects of sociological horror stories in the twentieth century.[80] In the nineteenth century, writers of advice on family relations approvingly encouraged men to give their wives greater influence over their children and to support maternal authority rather than to assert independently their own paternal power. If a father's assistance in childrearing must be dispensed with, he could at least be solicitous not to retard the work by disagreeing with his wife's government of the family. In one moment a thoughtless or indulgent papa, ignorant of the circumstances surrounding a conflict between mother and child, could overthrow the discipline that it had taken mama months to instill. The words, "My dear, do give the child what it wants" or "Wife, govern your own temper before you attempt to govern the child," spoken in the presence of children constituted domestic treason because they undermined a mother's authority. Father and mother must present a united front to their children, advisors warned, and unified parental authority meant enforcing maternal will with paternal strength.[81]

This constituted a remarkable theoretical shift in the power to legislate domestic life. The Americans who described the transfer of parental power from father to mother explicitly attributed the change to modern conditions of work, saying that if a father could not spend more than evenings and Sundays with his children, inevitably the task of discipline fell to the mother. Still, new material conditions alone cannot explain why or how the maternal role appreciated socially in modern America. A new respect for women's intellectual and moral strength supported the claims for maternal power. A developing ideology of women's moral superiority helped justify their responsibility for raising and educating children, and in turn, the gravity of that responsibility fueled the growing movement to improve educational opportunities for women themselves.

Before the mid-eighteenth century, Americans gave little thought to the issue of educating women; a sustained, systematic exchange of ideas on the subject, and the schools that testified to the relevance of the debate, appeared late in the century. The opening of private academies for women and the expansion of public school systems later in the nineteenth century represented a means for women to acquire a rudimentary education comparable to that of most men, but they also represented a concession, however imperfect, that women and men had fundamentally equal intellects.

This innovative and modern judgment is often slighted. When American educators first began to evaluate the nature of woman's intellectual capabilities, about 1800, they also considered the uses to which she might put her education. To these two separate questions educators usually provided two inherently incompatible answers, which they presented in theoretical essays and applied to the curriculum of schools. They maintained that women and men enjoyed equal intellects, yet also argued that knowledge should be used in sexually appropriate ways. Most educated women, as well as men, believed that women should apply their intellects to domestic or quasi-domestic problems. Even the women who earned college and advanced graduate degrees late in the nineteenth century created careers in service professions that had maternal nurturing qualities, such as social work and home economics.[82]

The contradictions in these judgments have played themselves out during the last century and a half, and we are becoming acutely conscious of the conflict between recognizing and training women's intellect and then confining the situations in which it is to be used. To do so is rather like attempting to power a bicycle with a jet engine—it creates a frustrating, wasteful, and inherently unstable combination. Yet our perception that advanced education has not "liberated" women from sex-typed social roles in the twentieth century should not blind us to the fact that, about 1800, American educators did begin to reevaluate woman's intellect. Furthermore, in the nineteenth century, the argument that developing women's minds would have domestic utility considerably enlarged women's opportunities to study. Only the domestic ends of women's education supposedly justified teaching them at all. And what now seem to be stale, conservative arguments designed to keep women devoted to home and family were considerably fresher and more liberal ideas in 1800.

As Mary Benson concluded in her survey of colonial American women, the radical thinkers in 1700 believed that women who had developed independent intellects through the study of history, literature, and languages would be better wives (and mothers). The few people who wrote these bold thoughts were English. Americans, and most English people, generally took a considerably narrower view— that women needed no education or only enough to pick their way through the Bible. As the century passed, more people conceded that teaching girls a few so-called accomplishments might enhance their value as marital companions or strengthen their morals.[83] God had "with the most conspicuous wisdom" discriminated between the mental powers of the two sexes, said Thomas Osborne, whose much-read essay on the duties of women summed up the conventional wisdom on the subject in the 1780s. Naturally, women could not comprehend any study or occupation that demanded close, comprehensive reasoning. But if they floundered helplessly in the study of law, philosophy, or commercial enterprise, women could comfortably navigate through such works of history, biography, and poetry as would improve their conversation and sense of virtue.[84]

Before 1780 most English girls' boarding schools had adopted a similarly limited approach to education. Particularly attractive to the daughters of merchants and wealthy farmers, the schools offered to transform girls into ladies by giving them instruction in needlework, music, drawing, and deportment, and practice in reading sermons. The first American academies for girls, which opened in cities after the Revolution, also catered to well-to-do families who could spare daughters to learn social graces. The object of education was clear to Alice Lee Shippen (wife of Dr. William Shippen), who encouraged her daughter Nancy to study diligently at Mrs. Rogers's Boarding School in 1777. "Tell me how you improve your work," mother inquired of

daughter. "Needlework is a most important branch of female education. How do you hold your head and shoulders, in making a curtsy,
in going out or coming into a room, in giving & receiving, holding
your knife & fork, walking seting."[85] Mrs. Rogers's education was designed to finish, not enlarge, the female intellect.

Private schools for women as well as men multiplied at the end of
the eighteenth century. Located in large cities and scattered gener-
ously throughout New England (which quickly became the academy
of America), the schools demonstrated republican enthusiasm for education. Though terms and graduation requirements were irregular and
classes were ungraded or of mixed ability, schools began to offer a
broader education to more girls, in reading and grammar as well as in
fundamentals of mathematics, geography, and history. Some of the
early private schools, such as the Young Ladies Academy that opened
in Philadelphia in 1787, thrived on the tuition paid by successful merchants. Others in lesser towns owed their tenuous life to gifts, public
subscriptions, and lotteries. A farm girl like Mary Lyon would earn
the right to study in exchange for sweeping out classrooms and assisting with teaching, a form of tuition that she later offered to her own
pupils at Mount Holyoke. Later, generally after 1800, free common
schools opened their doors to poorer girls.[86]

Enough girls attended private and public grammar schools and went
on to the secondary private academies that we can identify a generation of formally educated and publicly influential women by the early
years of the nineteenth century. Authors Lydia Huntley Sigourney
and Harriet Beecher Stowe learned to write essays in academy classrooms, as did abolitionists and suffragists such as Lucretia Coffin Mott
and Elizabeth Cady Stanton. Emma Willard, Mary Lyon, and Catharine Beecher emerged from New England schoolhouses convinced
of their mission to found schools and teach more women.[87] Hundreds
of their classmates did not achieve their eminence, yet gained a keener
sense of social or religious responsibility, the credentials to teach, or a
circle of friends from all over the country that they would maintain
for a lifetime.

There were, Maris Vinovskis and Richard Bernard remind us,
boundaries to women's educational experience. Girls were more likely
to attend schools in the Northeast, where general interest in education

ran high and school systems were better organized. Most girls went only a few terms to free common schools, not to private academies.[88] However, even though fewer girls than boys attended school, it is remarkable that so many women stepped within schoolrooms in so short a time. In eighteenth-century New England over half of all women could not sign their own names; by the 1840s most white women in America could read and write.[89] Some of the meaning of this accomplishment emerges in the painfully written letters of women informally educated in the eighteenth century. For these women, writing even a few lines was a great undertaking. Prefacing their correspondence with apologies for deficiences in spelling and composition, they urged their younger relatives to improve their writing.[90] With schooling, they knew, a woman could write legibly, correctly, and without shame.

A historic departure, this widespread extension of schooling to American girls meant in part that Americans had increased money and time to spend on women's education, but it also was the product of changing ideas about the utility of educating women. Liberal educators pronounced lessons in embroidery and etiquette of little practical or intellectual value, especially in the new republic. To manage their households, help their husbands, and raise their children competently, the arguments ran, American women needed more rigorous schooling. School administrators of secondary academies added courses in composition and mathematics to their curricula for women and later, in the nineteenth century, included physical sciences as well, in their attempts to produce disciplined women who could make a social contribution as mothers or teachers. These were vigorous ideas and innovations that made the educational goals of pre-Revolutionary Americans and the prescriptions of English writers Thomas Osborne and Hannah More appear conservative.[91]

Reform in American women's education was in some ways a consequence of the political changes of the early nineteenth century. The act of federating a republic inspired Americans to reflect on the value of education in their new nation and led some of them to advocate educational opportunities greater than those of Europe for women as well as men. The Revolution, explained educators, had enlarged the political significance of what women did in their homes and made it necessary to give them an appropriate education. Benjamin Rush established himself as an expert on the subject in 1787 by delivering his "Thoughts Upon Female Education" to the graduates of the Young Ladies Academy in Philadelphia. He enumerated the ways that informed women would strengthen the nation, declaring that the education of women should be adapted to the republican society in which they lived. Since Americans were so busy and their occupations so varied, women should be educated to help their husbands and assume the teaching of children. They should be able to read, write a legible hand, and know enough mathematics to keep their husbands' business accounts. The study of chemistry and natural philosophy would prevent supersitition and apply to culinary purposes, and a knowledge of history would enable them to instruct their sons in the principles of liberty and government. Rush recommended dropping courses in instrumental music and French because they took time from useful study; women had no time to practice the pianoforte. In short, systematic study of challenging subjects would produce self-reliant and reasonable, although domestic, women.[92]

Rush's contemporaries shared his opinion on the political value of educating women, as well as his conviction that women's contribution to public order was at best indirect. As Linda Kerber's review of their writings shows, no matter how sophisticated the intellectual underpinnings of their theories, Americans imagined women to be the silent partners in the republican compact, helpmeets of freemen, teachers of future citizens.[93]

The ideal of the educated mother proved a particularly attractive way for men and women to integrate domesticity and politics, and it was consequently a view frequently espoused by educators in the early nineteenth century. Catharine Beecher repeatedly and successfully solicited financial aid for women's academies by arguing that such contributions amounted to an investment in good government. Women might not "thunder from the forum" or make laws, but they "send forth the sages that govern and renovate the world."[94] The test of American schools, read another woman's variation on the argument, lay in the answer to the question, "Are American women qualified to educate the future men of our country?" In 1841 the answer was not a resounding affirmative, for she anticipated the happy day when "the intellectual women of our country formed a noble phalanx," able to promote the highest interests of their sex and guard the homes of the Republic.[95]

The political logic of maintaining that persons unable to vote and lacking citizenship were well qualified to teach lessons in citizenship is flimsy, and Beecher's position exasperated her contemporaries who asked for the right of direct political participation. Yet in a nation that preferred to listen to Daniel Webster say, innocent of irony, that mothers preserved free government by teaching their children that "the exercise of the elective franchise is a social duty, of as solemn nature as a man can be called to perform," the argument made sense and advanced women's opportunities to be educated.[96]

More realistic and more compelling were the promises that vigorous intellectual training would improve domestic life. If one considered education simply a process of accumulating information, the domestic consequences appeared gratifying. Immediate material benefits would come to homes where mistresses had studied chemistry and anatomy. Informed women would ventilate their houses properly, dress and feed their children healthfully. If only the housewives of Elizabethtown, Pennsylvania, had been familiar with the first principles of chemical science in 1814, they never would have stored their acid applesauce in red earthenware jars, and no one in that unfortunate community would have died of lead poisoning.[97] But intellectual life with a dull wife or mother could be dangerous too; it was, educators said, impossible for a woman to be a suitable companion and counselor with an uninformed mind and untutored heart. With a mind stored with the wisdom of the past and the literature of the day, she could converse thoughtfully with her husband and satisfy her children's need for knowledge. Their power "in the single relation of mother" justified educating women, Emma Willard reminded the New York legislature as she pleaded for its support in establishing an academy. "Would we rear the human plant to perfection, we must first fertilize the soil which produces it."[98]

Paradoxically, the growing emphasis on motherhood as women's greatest task in life, and the conviction of mothers' profound influence on their children, gave women more importance at the same time as it bound them more firmly to their homes. Their importance as mothers gave women more control over their homes and families, but it also helped to prevent any expansion of their influence outside their families; it offered a convincing argument for improving women's education while at the same time placing limits on the extent of their schooling. Perhaps most significantly, it created new respect for women and helped improve their status in society—but at the expense of inventing new reasons for limiting their participation in society. Just at the time when industrialization and the expansion of a market economy began to reduce women's domestic responsibilities and offer the possibility of employment outside the home, the elevation of motherhood to a divine calling created a whole new set of domestic responsibilities and new justifications for limiting women's influence to the narrow sphere of the family.

Toward the Twentieth Century: Changes in the Management of Birth and Motherhood

By the middle of the nineteenth century, childbirth had changed from a frequent event in women's lives, managed by other women, to an occasional event controlled by male physicians; and motherhood had been transformed from one of many domestic duties to the most critical task of most women's lives. Birth became an exceptional, rather than an ordinary, event. At the same time each child became a unique individual, demanding a mother's closest attention.

These two sets of changes—in the act of childbirth itself and in the lengthy process of childrearing—were inseparably linked. They affected women of different classes, ethnic backgrounds, and geographic regions at different times and to different degrees, but over the course of the nineteenth century virtually all American women felt their effects. As childbirth came to be viewed as an exceptional rather than a common event, each child took on greater significance; conversely, as mothering took on greater importance, women felt compelled to limit the number of children they bore. Bearing and rearing children ceased to be inevitable and natural and became events to be planned, studied, and controlled. Motherhood was no longer simply a woman's private concern but was a matter of public discussion and management.

The changes of the late eighteenth and early nineteenth centuries continued and expanded in the latter part of the nineteenth century and the early years of the twentieth. The average number of births per woman continued to decline, as the knowledge and practice of birth control became more sophisticated and widespread. Physicians continued to expand their control over childbirth, as they improved scientific methods of delivery, introduced anesthesia, and increasingly moved birth from the home into the hospital. And the general concern about the social importance of motherhood intensified. By the beginning of the twentieth century, social reformers took up the cause of motherhood as an issue of public debate and social legislation.

In all these ways Americans expressed the nineteenth century's growing concern with the importance of the individual and with man's mastery over nature. Just as Americans no longer accepted the inevitability of constant pregnancies and large families, so too they refused to accept informal or haphazard methods of delivering babies, high rates of infant and childhood mortality, or even the pain of childbirth. Faith in science, in the importance of the individual, and in man's power to improve his lot replaced an earlier age's stoical acceptance of the will of God and the ravages of nature.

The author of one pamphlet giving instructions on the prevention of conception summed up the prevailing wisdom of his age, saying that "the great Architect intended, that man should make use of his reasoning and inventive powers for the improvement of his station." Americans agreed, in biological as well as industrial matters, that giving instinct preference over reason would "drive the whole human family back to the woods for food and protection."[1] A full discussion of these changes would require another volume, but this chapter explores some of the kinds of changes that resulted from the transformation of motherhood into woman's sacred mission.

For centuries, many women had attempted to limit the number of their pregnancies by abstinence, withdrawal, prolonged nursing of infants, as well as by various folk methods of dubious efficacy. But by the mid-nineteenth century family limitation became both more prevalent and more socially acceptable. The open dissemination of birth control information and devices remained a subject of controversy until well into the twentieth century; but the practice of birth control nevertheless won increasing acceptance among middle-class American couples in the nineteenth century. The national decline in the fertility rate of white American women, which began around the beginning of the century, continued steadily into the twentieth; whereas a colonial woman could expect to carry eight pregnancies, a white urban woman of 1910 carried an average of five. The gradual decline in the birthrate was a direct consequence of widespread acceptance of the practice of birth control.[2]

Histories of contraception have emphasized the public campaigns of the late nineteenth and early twentieth centuries and have often assumed that there was a little contraceptive information available in the mid-nineteenth century. In fact, however, such information was extensive in the earlier decades of the century; the anti–birth control legislation and purity campaigns of the late nineteenth century were in large part a response to increasing popular use of birth control. Newspaper and magazine advertisements promising cures for "womb troubles" or "female irregularities," or offering "preventative pessaries," "shields," and "hygenic syringes" for sale offer some clues about the sources of birth control information. Women also learned from private letters and public lectures on hygiene and from pamphlets and books on medicine directed to young women specifically.[3]

Literature specifically about birth control, which advanced the argument that men and women ought to consider the importance of motherhood before deciding to conceive a child, was first published in the United States by the third decade of the nineteenth century. The first book on birth control to appear in America was Robert Dale Owen's *Moral Physiology*, published in New York in 1830. Owen, son of the well-known English social reformer, used the need to control population growth as his primary argument in favor of family limitation, but he also urged the importance of birth control to preserve the health of women and to ensure that couples had only as many children as they could support comfortably. His fact book was an attempt to persuade couples to limit their families, rather than a medical handbook on birth control methods; his preferred method was withdrawal, and he warned couples that chemical and mechanical devices were ineffective. *Moral Physiology*, despite its limitations, was enormously popular; 75,000 copies of it were sold in the United States and England by the time of Owen's death in 1877.[4]

Charles Knowlton, a Massachusetts physician, was more specific about the medical details of contraception in his book, *The Fruits of Philosophy*, published originally in England in 1832. Knowlton recommended douching with any one of a variety of preparations, ranging from solutions of alum, rose leaves, green tea, zinc sulfate, or sugar of lead to ordinary baking soda.[5] Knowlton's methods apparently enjoyed considerable popularity. Far from being gratified, Knowlton was distressed that he did not receive more credit for his ideas. Claiming that he had originated douching as a contraceptive, he argued that subsequent publications mentioning his method were an infringement of his copyright.[6] *The Fruits of Philosophy* remained an influential work for several decades; it went through numerous editions, with the later ones considerably edited and expanded by others.

Knowlton's book, the first of its kind in the United States, was followed by a series of similar publications, written by physicians or by other men claiming the title of "doctor" without benefit of degree, or by lecturers in phrenology or hygiene. Their books gave information on a variety of contraceptive techniques, ranging from the use of douches, sponges, condoms, and diaphragms, to sexual abstinence during the fertile period, to total continence.

The rationale for birth control in this early literature is not predominantly Malthusian (notwithstanding Owen's comments on the potential danger of overpopulation), nor was it eugenic, as was often the case later in the century. The arguments were highly personal, rather than abstractly social; most of the books used letters from patients and case histories to link arguments for birth control firmly to the problems of families, and particularly women, with too many children. Primarily concerned with the health, status, and duties of women, they offered definitions of the meaning of motherhood not previously expressed in America. The ideas were not the property of any faction of suffragists or "free love" groups, though they supported what has come to be identified as women's rights and therefore can be construed loosely as "feminist."

The general nature of the birth control literature is reflected in the case histories that speak of woman per se; of women who are feeble and unfit to fulfill their family duties during pregnancy; and of women constitutionally unable to bear children, for whom, in the language of one of the pamphlets, sexual intercourse is a "death wound."[7] The material deplores the fate of women married young and doomed to be old at thirty because of frequent childbearing. The manuals advise intervals of two to four years between each pregnancy so that the mother will have a chance to recover her health and each child will receive proper attention.

The message of the literature was not restricted to women. The pamphlets speak to men too, telling them that "no man ought to require or expect that the whole life of an intellectual, refined, and cultivated female should be spent in bringing into the world, and raising through infancy and childhood, a family of twelve or fifteen children."[8] Some authors of birth control literature argued that a continually pregnant woman would come to hate her husband for ruining her health and burdening her life, and would also hate her unwanted children. Henry C. Wright wrote of the "Crime of Undesired Maternity" that deprived women of their right to decide when they wanted to be pregnant. Women should not have children, one doctor warned, "Unless it is her express wish." For her husband, "her feelings, her interests should be *imperative* law."[9]

These observations have a variety of implications. They argue, obviously, for a growing public awareness of the intricate relation between procreation and pleasure; for the separation of procreation and pleasure is the underlying premise of any form of contraception other than abstinence. However, more germane for the argument at hand, they state that woman's willing participation is vital in the sex act because she must consider what motherhood will mean to her before she conceives a child, even before marriage. As one man exhorted, "Maidens, never enter into the physical relations of marriage with a man until you have conversed with him freely and fully on maternity. Learn his expectations in regard to that purest and most enobling of all the functions of your nature." He warned women not to be "victimized" by a man who will not control his passions and would turn them into "weak, miserable, unlovable and degraded wives and mothers" by disregarding contraception.[10]

The importance of motherhood and of the individuality of children demanded some form of family limitation—clearly, women could not live up to the ideals of motherhood expected of them in the nineteenth century and still raise as many children as their colonial sisters had done. And yet, the power to control pregnancy also offered women the potential for much greater independence, even for total release from the duties of motherhood. These implications became increasingly apparent to women and men in the second half of the nineteenth century. To many people, the dangers of birth control far outweighed its advantages; ironically, as information about contraception became more readily available, campaigns to outlaw such information intensified. Opponents of birth control focused most often on the supposed moral depravity that would result from the separation of sex and procreation; but, by implication, they also deplored the possibility that contraception might change women's traditional role as wife and mother.

The reprinting of Knowlton's *Fruits of Philosophy* in England in 1877 brought criminal charges against Charles Bradlaugh and Annie Besant, who had sponsored its publication.[11] One of the ironies of the anti–birth control movement, however, was the fact that the publicity it generated served only to spread knowledge of contraceptive methods. By the century's end, well before Margaret Sanger's highly publicized crusades, the practice of birth control, through contraception and abortion, was familiar to many American women.[12] When Dr. John King wryly reported to his colleagues in the Riverside County Medical Society in 1899 that "most up-to-date young women, encumbered with husbands, can furnish an epitome of means and methods" of contraception, he echoed reports of physicians throughout the country.[13] In professional journals they related the contraceptive advice that they gave to women and argued that their advice was justified when childbirth would be emotionally or physically dangerous for the mother.

Such arguements for contraception contain the recognition that women are meant to live their lives beyond a continual state of pregnancy, emphasizing that childrearing, rather than childbearing, is woman's most important social task. They demonstrated, often explicitly, that Americans used reason and science to control the natural rate of human reproduction.

As women increasingly controlled the frequency of pregnancy, so too physicians worked to control the conditions of childbirth. They accomplished this control by increasing use of surgical instruments; by administering anesthesia to diminish or even eliminate the pain of childbirth; and finally, toward the end of the nineteenth century, by taking birth out of the home altogether and moving it into the hospital.

American doctors first employed ether and chloroform to relieve birth pain in 1848. Walter Channing, a Boston physician who was the first American to use anesthesia, urged other physicians to administer the new drugs on humanitarian grounds. They had the power to eliminate pain, he argued.[14] Not all doctors were certain about the safety of ether and chloroform, however; nor were all convinced that women ought to have their labor pains alleviated. The possibility of using the drugs prompted physicians, clergymen, and women to publish exhaustive arguments on the moral and medical responsibility of physicians to control birth pain. By 1900 obstetrical anesthesia was common, particularly in cases where doctors used instruments. Some were concerned about potential danger to mother and child if anesthesia was employed. But moral arguments were more common than medical arguments. Birth pain was part of the curse of Eve, and mere mortals should not try to eliminate it, many men argued. More popular was the belief that the pain of labor and childbirth strengthened the love of a mother for her child.[15] Women, understandably, were eager to find ways to ease the suffering of childbirth, and so the use of anesthesia became a subject of considerable controversy during the second half of the nineteenth century. The use of anesthesia remained relatively uncommon, however, until the twentieth century; when drugs were employed, they were used to dull pain rather than to produce complete unconsciousness.

Uncertainty about the potential dangers of anesthesia and moral arguments against it combined to limit its use in the nineteenth century. After World War I, however, new techniques along with the increasing tendency for women to deliver their babies in hospitals (where anesthesia was more easily administered) encouraged more frequent use of painkilling drugs. "Twilight sleep," as the new anesthesia came to be called, was first developed in Germany. Initially rejected by American doctors as unsafe, it became widely used by the 1920s and 1930s after several women, led by woman physicians, mounted a campaign to have the new method adopted in American hospitals. A Boston physician, Eliza Taylor Ransom, established a maternity hospital in 1914 for the purpose of delivering babies using twilight sleep; she also formed the New England Twilight Sleep Association. Largely as a result of her efforts, all Boston hospitals employed the new procedures by the early 1920s. By the late 1930s, it was used in most hospital births.[16]

The twilight sleep method began with an injection of morphine when the expectant mother first went into labor. A dose of scapalomine, a hallucinogenic drug that induces amnesia, followed. This combination of drugs not only dulled pain but also made women completely unaware of birth. As many physicians suspected, twilight sleep was a dangerous procedure, because it prevented women from actually participating in birth and could harm their infants. But women, eager to be freed from the pain of childbirth, hailed the new anesthesia as the final liberation of woman from the curse of Eve and demanded use of the new techniques. Perhaps more than anything else, these techniques induced women to have their babies in hospitals.

Medical control of birth improved the conditions of childbearing and the mother's chances of survival in some ways, but it created new problems and dangers as well. Physicians who had general surgical practices carried puerperal infections with them to their obstetrical cases, increasing the death toll from childbed fever. Oliver Wendell Holmes, observing the pattern of outbreaks of puerperal fever among Boston women, concluded in 1843 that doctors transmitted contagion to their patients. Even when doctors were willing to accept that they carried pestilence, and took antiseptic measures against an undefined and invisible enemy, the fever was extraordinarily persistent. Identifying and controlling puerperal fever troubled doctors well into the twentieth century. Fear of sepsis justified managing birth under sterile conditions, like a surgical procedure.

Ultimately, this concern with maintaining antiseptic conditions at birth, and with the scientific management of childbirth in general, encouraged physicians to conduct increasing numbers of deliveries in hospitals rather than in patients' homes. In doing so, they completed the transformation of birth from a private, exclusively female experience into a male-controlled "illness."

The transfer of birth from home to hospital was the most significant

change in American customs of childbirth during the fifty years between 1870 and 1920. As was the case with earlier changes in childbirth customs, this shift occurred first in large cities, primarily in the
eastern part of the country.

Only about 5 percent of American women delivered in hospitals in
1900, but by 1920 the figures ranged from 30 percent in Philadelphia
to 65 percent in San Francisco, the city with the highest proportion
of hospital maternity cases in the country.[17] Most of these births occurred in hospitals established specifically to treat women, some of them
exclusively for maternity cases. The histories of these hospitals are remarkably similar. All began as small, private charities for destitute
women. They opened in converted residences and took in patients referred by attending physicians and reputable boardinghouse keepers
or brought in by policemen. Physicians donated their services, and
visiting medical students worked for clinical experience. In the case of
at least one hospital in every city, woman doctors organized the hospitals to provide reciprocal medical care and experience for their own
sex.

Until the twentieth century, the overwhelming majority of patients
in maternity hospitals were foreign-born, or native single women. Because of the low social status of the patients, the hospitals at times had
difficulty distinguishing themselves from the pestilent public alms-
houses and from the so-called lying-in hospitals that were in reality
abortion mills. By the outset of the twentieth century all the hospitals
had gathered enough support to construct special, large hospital
buildings, and had medical and social reputations acceptable to respectable middle-class women.

The hospital provided an arena in which for several groups of city
people might work. The medical staff, which became highly conscious of the training value of the institutions, was only one part of
the hospital administration. The newly rich, who sought some way to
contribute to their city and confirm their status in monumental fashion, donated large sums of money to building funds. In this manner,
for example, Phoebe Apperson Hearst associated herself with Children's Hospital in San Francisco, and J. Pierpont Morgan identified
with the Lying-in Hospital of New York. Another group, primarily
women wealthy in time rather than in money, composed the auxili-

aries of every hospital, which sponsored endless rounds of bazaars, solicited donations from merchants, hemmed sheets, and frequently paid
home visits to discharged patients.

These men and women who created medical charities recognized a
great urban social problem in feminine terms. They provided care for
destitute women in cities, "in the most critical hour of woman's need."[18]
They expressed their mission in the same terms as the attending physician of the New England Hospital for Women did in 1865, when
she wrote that her hospital was "a necessity in a city like Boston." It
served the wives of transients so common in a great city; it gave de-
cent care to women unwilling to go to the common poorhouse; and it
saved unmarried women "from physical and moral ruin."[19]

By the turn of the century, hospital administrators thought that they
had a special responsibility to immigrant women in the city. They came
to link the benefits of hospital care with superior American values. The
midwives who advertised their trade in German throughout New York,
argued the staff of the New York Lying-in Hospital, were ignorant of
antiseptic treatment of childbirth. The safest delivery was possible only
in circumstances where the physician could employ sterile techniques
and new technology.[20]

By the 1920s, however, it was no longer only immigrant and pov-
erty-stricken women who went to hospitals to give birth. Increasing
numbers of middle-class women also came to believe that the controlled environment of the hospital was safer than the home for childbirth. In fact, the maternity hospitals eventually became largely the
province of white middle- and upper-class women rather than of the
poor and immigrant mothers for whom they were originally intended.
Old World cultural practices died hard; the immigrant women who
were the targets of well-meaning doctors and social reformers preferred to employ midwives, often from their own ethnic backgrounds,
until well into the twentieth century.

There were a number of reasons for native-born, middle-class
women's increasing preference for hospital births. Puerperal fever
continued to be a danger, and both women and doctors believed that
the antiseptic conditions of the hospital offered the best protection
against fever. More sophisticated methods of anesthesia were best administered under hospital conditions. And nonmedical considerations

had an influence too; smaller homes and fewer servants made it more difficult to care for convalescents at home. The hotel-like conditions of the hospital catered to urban families who could no longer rely on relatives, neighbors, and servants to care for a new mother and her baby for an extended period of time.

One of the consequences of the scientific management of childbirth was to isolate women in labor and delivery from their families, friends, and the familiar surroundings of their homes. For each individual woman, childbirth became an intensely private experience. On the abstract level, however, childbirth became a public issue—a subject for the crusades of social reformers and the debates of legislators. Establishing hospitals for indigent women and trying to persuade immigrants to give up their midwives had been an early manifestation of public concern with childbearing and motherhood; that concern intensified and broadened in the early decades of the twentieth century, as social reformers donated much of their attention to protecting the lives and well-being of women and children.

Some of their programs, such as the pensions given to widowed and abandoned mothers to maintain their families, crystallized in statute form social ideals of a mother's importance in family life. Other reforms, such as the Supreme Court ruling on women's working hours in 1908, recognized the rights of women who worked outside their homes, away from their families, yet offered special protection on the grounds that "women's physical structure and the performance of maternal functions place her at a disadvantage." It was in the public interest to "preserve the strength and vigor of the race" by preserving the health of women.[21]

During the years between 1880 and 1930, public and private agencies created a variety of programs specifically designed to promote the health of childbearing women and to lower the death rate from causes related to pregnancy. By 1930 maternal welfare was an established department function in the majority of large American cities, and agents of federal and state programs were working to help mothers in rural areas. These programs were by no means comprehensive, but the line of developing policy was clear. Government now added its weight to that of the medical profession in promoting the management of childbirth.

Maternal health programs were designed to lower the unusually high rate of American maternal mortality. A Bureau of the Census report of 1906 first called attention to the high rate of maternal and child death. In 1912 the federal government established the Children's Bureau to oversee issues concerning the health and welfare of mothers and children. Its first task was to study the incidence and causes of infant and maternal mortality. The Children's Bureau studies revealed that the United States had among the highest rates of infant and maternal mortality in the industrialized world. In 1916 more than 16,000 mothers died from childbirth, a higher death rate than any "principal country" but Spain or Switzerland, and this figure increased to 23,000 in 1918.[22] Appalled, reformers called this statistic a blot on the United States, one "greater than war losses," and pointed out that it "did not require a very constructive imagination" to comprehend the economic loss from these casualties or the "suffering, broken homes, and the grief of motherless children."[23] The high rate of maternal mortality also caused alarm because it was coupled with a declining birthrate.

Those who studied the causes of the problem found a high correlation between poverty and maternal death rates, but providing an adequate income for the families of childbearing women was a political impossibility. Instead, reformers devoted their attention to three other contributing agents—midwives, patients, and physicians—and created programs to regulate the medical profession, improve the training of doctors, and educate childbearing women in the hygiene of pregnancy.

Predictably, the midwife attracted a generous share of blame for deaths in childbirth. Although reformers recognized that she provided cheap obstetrical service to immigrants, professionally she was "only a makeshift."[24] The prevailing sentiment, especially among woman physicians, was that untrained, the midwife was dangerous, and if allowed to practice with a minimum of training, she lowered the standards of the profession. New York City, in which midwives delivered over half the children in 1900, created the first and most comprehensive system of regulation, obtaining a midwives' licensing law from the state legislature in 1907. Other cities, including Boston, outlawed midwives. Some southern states initiated training programs for black midwives.

Reformers regulated midwives, but they sought to educate their potential patients about the importance of proper diet and hygiene throughout pregnancy and proper sanitary conditions at birth. Programs of education and medical care proliferated as hospitals instituted maternity clinics. Cities hired nurses to supervise low-income women during pregnancy and to visit them after their deliveries. The federal Children's Bureau circulated pamphlets about prenatal care and distributed funds to states for visiting nurses, consultation centers, and conferences on childbirth until the provisions of the Sheppard Towner Act of 1921.

Under scrutiny, the history of the Sheppard Towner Act appears similar to that of other Progressive legislative reforms. It is a record of clashes between reformers' ideals and physicians' self-interests, and of compromise produced by fear of creating too many legislative restrictions on private activity. The American Medical Association, for example, which might have been expected to support the bill because it encouraged professional care during childbirth, rejected it because it might lead to socialized medicine. (In the late 1920s pressure from physicians finally forced an end to the funding of programs established under the act.) What emerges clearly, however, is the importance of women as physicians and public health professionals, and as a general lobby, in creating pressure to pass the bill. And the act did indicate a definite commitment to improve the welfare of women.

These programs of maternal health, though limited and unsystematic, affected the management of childbearing. They did not, on the whole, reduce the rate of maternal mortality, but they did recognize the dimensions of the problem and declare that the city, state, and federal governments had an obligation to women. The Sheppard Towner Act in particular aroused great public interest in maternity, teaching women what to ask for and what to expect from doctors. On the whole, the programs emphasized the importance of having trained medical professionals manage childbirth. The educational programs stressed the need for continuous care throughtout pregnancy, historically a novelty, which also strengthened medical involvement in childbirth.

By 1930 the patterns of modern American childbearing and childrearing were clear. In 200 years the life cycle of American women had changed greatly. Before 1800, being a mother meant being primarily a childbearer; but by the third decade of the twentieth century, pregnancy was increasingly an isolated event in women's lives, and being a mother meant rearing children more than bearing them.

The campaigns of Margaret Sanger and her associates had made it possible for highly motivated women of all socioeconomic groups to obtain reliable contraceptive services; as a result, a substantial number of American women were using some method of birth control. Well-educated, urban, Protestant women averaged only slightly more than one birth per woman.[25] Childbirth itself became more than ever a medical rather than a social event, as more women went to hospitals to deliver their babies and doctors refined their obstetrical techniques. Surgical intervention became increasingly common; in some hospitals doctors used forceps in one-quarter to one-half of all births and resorted to caesarian section in a substantial number of cases. And with increasing medical complexity came higher costs for pregnancy and birth. Many young couples felt compelled to consider the costs, as well as the responsibilities, of bearing children in making their decisions about raising a family. "Doctor, $200.00, Hospital, $192.00, Nurse, $192.00, Operating Room, $20.00, Incidentals, $50.00 = $654.00" was the discouraging total that confronted those who wanted good maternity care in 1929.[26] Some people asserted that it was high enough to deter the educated middle class from having children.

Ironically, as motherhood gained importance as women's all-consuming occupation, their careers as mothers became shorter. Throughout the nineteenth century and into the twentieth, as birthrates declined and life expectancy increased, women completed both their childbearing and childrearing years at earlier ages.

"At the present day," Dorothy Fisher observed in 1941, "maternity is not the occupation of a lifetime. What are we going to do when we are grandmothers?"[27] This new problem of middle-aged mothers without children would disturb Fisher's daughters and would ultimately produce a reevaluation of the mother's role in American society.

Notes

INTRODUCTION

1. Abigail Adams to Mercy Otis Warren, July 16, 1773; Mercy Otis Warren to Abigail Adams, July 25, 1773, in *Adams Family Correspondence*, ed. Lyman H. Butterfield et al. (Cambridge, Mass., 1963, 1973), 1 : 85–86.

2. James Fordyce, *Sermons to Young Women* (Boston, 1767), 1 : 25.

3. Edmund S. Morgan, *The Puritan Family: Religion and Domestic Relations in Seventeenth Century New England*, rev. ed. (New York, 1966), 76–78.

4. See especially Mary Beth Norton, *Liberty's Daughters: The Revolutionary Experience of American Women, 1750–1800* (Boston, 1980), and, on women's education in particular, Linda K. Kerber, *Women of the Republic: Intellect and Ideology in Revolutionary America* (Chapel Hill, N.C., 1980).

5. To John Adams, March 31, 1776, in Butterfield et al., *Adams Family Correspondence*, 1 : 370.

CHAPTER I

1. Benjamin Colman, *Some of the Honours that Religion Does Unto the Fruitful Mothers in Israel . . .* (Boston, 1715), 5, 7.

2. Laurel Thatcher Ulrich, *Good Wives: Image and Reality in the Lives of Women in Northern New England, 1650–1750* (New York, 1982), 159.

3. Julia Cherry Spruill, *Women's Life and Work in the Southern Colonies* (1938; reprint Chapel Hill, N.C., 1972), 45–46.

4. Benjamin Franklin, "Observations Concerning the Increase of Mankind, Peopling of Countries, Etc., Written in Pennsylvania, 1751," in *The Writings of Benjamin Franklin*, ed. Albert Henry Smyth (New York, 1907), 3 : 63–73; Thomas Malthus, *An Essay on the Principle of Population, as It Affects the Future Improvement of Society* (1798; reprint Baltimore, 1970), 73–74, 105–106. On colonial American population growth in general see Wilson H. Grabhill, Clyde V. Kiser, and Pascal K. Whelpton, "A Long View," in *The*

American Family in Social-Historical Perspective, ed. Michael Gordon (New York, 1973), 375–377; J. Potter, "The Growth of Population in America, 1700–1860," in *Population in History, Essays in Historical Demography* ed. David V. Glass and David E. C. Eversley (Chicago, 1965), 631–633, 643–644.

5. Arthur W. Calhoun, *A Social History of the American Family* (1917; reprint New York, 1960), 1 : 87.

6. John Demos, *A Little Commonwealth: Family Life in Plymouth Colony* (New York, 1970), 68; Grabhill, Kiser, and Whelpton, "A Long View," 374–383; Philip J. Greven, Jr., *Four Generations: Population, Land, and Family in Colonial Andover* (Ithaca, N.Y., 1970), 104–105, 202; Potter, "Growth of Population in America," 644, 647, 663, 679; Robert Wells, "Demographic Change and the Life Cycle of American Families," in *The Family in History: Interdisciplinary Essays*, ed. Theodore K. Rabb and Robert I. Rotberg (New York, 1971), 85, 88; Robert V. Wells, "Family Size and Fertility Control in Eighteenth-Century America, a Study of Quaker Families," *Population Studies* 25 (March 1971): 75–76. The average number of births, by nature, masks fluctuations within, and between, communities. Some of the specific figures are: Andover, Massachusetts, from 1660 to 1720—average births diminish from 8.3 to 7.6 per family (Greven, *Four Generations*); Plymouth, Old Colony, 8 or 9 per family (Demos, *Little Commonwealth*); Philadelphia Quakers, 1775, 6.68 per family (Wells, "Demographic Change").

7. Grabhill, Kiser, and Whelpton, "Long View," 374–384; Potter, "Growth of Population," 631–633, 643–644.

8. Franklin, "Observations Concerning the Increase of Mankind," *Writings of Benjamin Franklin*, 63–65; Malthus, *An Essay*, 73–74, 104–105.

9. Grabhill, Kiser, and Whelpton, "Long View," 383–388; Potter, "Growth of Population," 663; Maris A. Vinovkis, "Socioeconomic Determinants of Interstate Fertility Differentials in the United States in 1850 and 1860," *Journal of Interdisciplinary History* 6 (Winter 1976): 375–396; Yasukichi Yasuba, *Birth Rates of the White Population in the United States, 1800–1860: An Economic Study* (Baltimore, 1962), 137–187.

10. Greven, *Four Generations*, 34–35, 120–121; Potter, "Growth of Population," 651, 663.

11. Robert H. Bremner, ed., *Children and Youth in America: A Documentary History, Volume I: 1600–1685* (Cambridge, Mass., 1970), 103–122, 145–169; Calhoun, *Social History of the American Family*, 124–127; Spruill, *Women's Life and Work*, 46. Quotation from Calhoun.

12. Colman, *Some of the Honours that Religion Does*, 6; Cotton Mather, *Elizabeth in Her Holy Retirement. An Essay to Prepare a Pious Woman for her Lying-in . . .* (Boston, 1710), 5; Benjamin Wadsworth, *The Well-Ordered Family: or, Relative Duties* (Boston, 1712), 100. Quotation from Wadsworth.

13. Journal of William Allason, cited in Wyndham B. Blanton, *Medicine in Virginia in the Eighteenth Century* (Richmond, Va., 1931), 25. For similar sentiments see William Byrd, *The Secret Diary of William Byrd of Westover, 1709–1712*, ed. Louis B. Wright and Marion Tinling (Richmond, Va., 1941), 142, 186; Calhoun, *Social History of the American Family*, 87; Samuel Sewall, *Diary of Samuel Sewall*, Massachusetts Historical Society Collections, 5th ser., vols. 5–7 (1878–1882), 5 : 56, 426; Spruill, *Women's Life and Work*, 47.

14. Greven, *Four Generations*, 187–190 196–197; Potter, "Growth of Population," 644, 659–660, 678–679; Richard H. Shryock, *Medicine and Society in America, 1660–1860* (Ithaca, N.Y., 1960), 99; Benjamin Franklin, "Increase of Mankind," p. 65.

15. Ansley J. Coale and Melvin Zelnik, *New Estimates of Fertility and Population in the United States: A Study of Annual White Births from 1855 to 1960 and of Completedness of Enumeration in the Census from 1880 to 1960* (Princeton, N.J., 1963), 35; David E. C. Eversley, *Social Theories of Fertility and the Malthusian Debate* (1958: reprint Westport, Conn., 1975), 283–284; Vinovkis, "Socioeconomic Determinants," 393, 396; Yasuba, *Birth Rates of White Population*, 187.

16. William and Malleville Haller, "The Puritan Art of Love," *Huntington Library Quarterly* 5 (January 1942): 242, 265–266; John T. Noonan, Jr., *Contraception: A History of Its Treatment by the Catholic Theologians and Canonists* (Cambridge, Mass., 1966), 303–340, 353; Robert V. Schnucker, "Elizabethan Birth Control and Puritan Attitudes," *Journal of Interdisciplinary History* 4 (Spring 1975): 660–667.

17. John Oliver, *A Present for Teeming American Women* (Boston, 1694), 6; Schnucker, "Elizabethan Birth Control," 660–664.

18. Colman, *Some of the Honours that Religion Does*, 5, 15; Mather, *Elizabeth in Her Holy Retirement*, 5; Oliver, *A Present for Teeming American Women*, 28.

19. Mather, *Elizabeth in Her Holy Retirement*, 4; Cotton Mather, *Ornaments for the Daughters of Zion, or the Character and Happiness of a Woman*, 3d ed. (Boston, 1741), 2–3. Colman, *Some of the Honours that Religion Does*, 7.

20. Colman, *Some of the Honours that Religion Does*, 8, 17; 1 Timothy 2 : 15; Mather, *Elizabeth in Her Holy Retirement*, 3; See also Schnucker, "Elizabethan Birth Control," 665.

21. Mather, *Elizabeth in Her Holy Retirement*, 3.

22. American editions of *Aristotle's Master Piece*, 1766, 1788, discussed in Otho T. Beall, Jr., "*Aristotle's Master Piece* in America: A Landmark in the Folklore of Medicine," *William and Mary Quarterly*, 3d ser., 20 (1963); 216.

23. Jack P. Greene, ed., *The Diary of Colonel Landon Carter of Sabine Hall, 1752–1788* (Charlottesville., Va., 1965), 2 : 713.

24. [Thomas Clap], "Memoirs of a College President; Womanhood in Early America," ed. Edwin Stanley Wells, *The Connecticut Magazine* 12 (1908): 236.

25. Cecil K. Drinker, *Not So Long Ago: A Chronicle of Medicine and Doctors in Colonial Philadelphia* (New York, 1937), 48.

26. Colman, *Some of the Honours that Religion Does*, 9, 17.

27. Robert V. Wells, "Family Size and Fertility Control in Eighteenth-Century America," *Population Studies* 25 (1971): 77–79. The average age of the mother at the birth of her last child is an index of the use of deliberate fertility control. Couples who limit the size of their families tend to have their children in the early years of their marriage.

28. William Langer, "Infanticide: A Historical Survey," *History of Childhood Quarterly* 1 (Winter 1974): 358–360; Edward A. Wrigley, "Family Limitation in Pre-Industrial England," in *Population in Industrialization*, ed. Michael Drake (London, 1969), 157–194.

29. Daniel Defoe, *Conjugal Lewdness, or Matrimonial Whoredom. A Treatise Concerning the Use and Abuse of the Marriage Bed* (1727; reprint London, 1967), 149–155; Noonan, *Contraception: A History*, 200–230, 342–344, 350; Schnucker, "Elizabethan Birth Control," 656–659.

30. Spruill, *Women's Life and Work*, 325–326.

31. Greene, *Diary of Carter* 2 : 859, 861.

32. Drinker, *Not So Long Ago*, 55, 59; Greene, *Diary of Carter* 1 : 511, 514; Robert G. Potter et al., "Applications of Field Studies to Research on the Physiology of Human Reproduction, Lactation and Its Effects upon Birth Intervals in Eleven Punjab

Villages, India," *Journal of Chronic Diseases* 18 (November 1965): 1125–1140; Christopher Tietze, "The Effect of Breastfeeding on the Rate of Conception," *International Population Conference Proceedings* 2 (1961): 129–136.

33. Colman, *Some of the Honours that Religion Does*, 9, 18; Mather, *Ornaments*, 99–100.

34. Wright and Tinling, *Diary of William Byrd*, 548; *Oxford English Dictionary*, s.v. "breeding"; Mitford M. Mathews, ed., *A Dictionary of Americanisms on Historical Principles* (Chicago, 1951), s.v. "breeding." "Teeming," also considered archaic dialect by the *OED*, applied to women from the sixteenth through the eighteenth centuries.

35. Linda Grant De Pauw and Conover Hunt, *Remember the Laies: Women in America, 1750–1815* (New York, 1976), 22 (photograph of dress in the Philadelphia Museum of Art), 24; Blanche Payne, *History of Costume from the Ancient Egyptians to the Twentieth Century* (New York, 1965), 413; pregnant women in foreground (pl. III, "Evening") in series *The Four Times of Day* by William Hogarth (1738), in *Engravings by Hogarth*, ed. Sean Shesgreen (New York, 1973), pl. 44; Estelle Ansley Worrell, *Early American Costume* (Harrisburg, Pa., 1975), 63, 68.

36. Payne, *History of Costume*, 416; Spruill, *Women's Life and Work*, 116–117; Worrell, *Early American Costume*, 31, 47, 63–64, 67.

37. Spruill, *Women's Life and Work*, 117; Worrell, *Early American Costume*, 63, 73.

38. Mary Vial Holyoke, diary, in *The Holyoke Diaries, 1709–1856*, ed., George Francis Dow (Salem, Mass., 1911), 48, 58, 70; Edward Augustus Holyoke, MS, description of midwife bungling delivery about 1763, written 1783, MS, Holmes Hall, Countway Collection, Harvard Medical School Library; Sewall, *Diary* 6 : 50; Francis G. Wallett, ed., "The Diary of Ebenezer Parkman, 1729–1738," *Proceedings of the American Antiquarian Society* 71, pt. 2 (October 18, 1961), 441–442.

39. Nicholas Culpeper, *A Directory for Midwives: or, A Guide for Women, in Their Conception, Bearing and Suckling their Children, Enlarged* (London, 1701), 278–286.

40. Charles Andrews, *Colonial Folkways* (New Haven, 1919), 147; Otho T. Beall, Jr., and Richard H. Shryock, *Cotton Mather, First Significant Figure in American Medicine* (Baltimore, 1954), 14; William G. Rothstein, *American Physicians in the Nineteenth Century: From Sects to Science* (Baltimore, 1972), 26–38; Shryock, *Medicine and Society in America*, 3–9.

41. Irving S. Cutter and Henry R. Viets, *A Short History of Midwifery* (Philadelphia, 1964), 4–10; Isaac Harvey Flack (pseud. Harvey Graham), *Eternal Eve* (London, 1950), 139, 176, 222–223, 226–231.

42. Shryock, *Medicine and Society in America*, 48–54; Richard H. Shryock, *Medicine in America: Historical Essays* (Baltimore, 1966), 4–11; Rothstein, *American Physicians*, 27.

43. Michael K. Eshleman, "Diet During Pregnancy in the Sixteenth and Seventeenth Centuries," *Journal of the History of Medicine* 30 (January 1975): 25–31.

44. Culpeper, *A Directory for Midwives* (London, 1651 edition), 55, 64–71, 79; Cutter and Viets, *Short History*, 11–15; Flack, *Eternal Eve*, 226–228. The Harvard Medical School Library catalog lists fourteen editions of Culpeper's *Directory* between 1651 and 1755.

45. Aristotle (pseud.), *Aristotle's Compleat and Experienc'd Midwife, in two Parts. I. Guide for Childbearing Women. II. Proper and Safe Remedies for the Curing of all those Distempers that are incident to the Female Sex . . .* , 9th ed. (London, [1700?]), 27; Culpeper, *A Directory for Midwives* (1701), 278–279; Eshleman, "Diet During Pregnancy," 26–28, 30–35; Jane Sharp, *The Compleat Midwife's Companion: or, the art of midwifery improved . . .* , 4th ed. (London, 1725), 112. Quotation from Sharp.

46. Culpeper, *A Directory for Midwives* (1701), 286; Thomas R. Forbes, *The Midwife*

and the Witch (New Haven, 1966), 64–71, 78–79 (see Chapter 5, pp. 61–79, on minerals and obstetrical amulets); Cotton Mather, *The Angel of Bethesda*, ed. Gordon W. Jones (Barre, Mass., 1972), 247; Sharp, *Compleat Midwife's Companion*, 112. Quotation from Sharp.

47. Mather, *The Angel of Bethesda*, 246; Sharp, *Compleat Midwife's Companion*, 112; Percival Willughby, *Observations in Midwifery*, Henry Blenkinsop (Wakefield, England, 1972 [orig. pub. 1803]), 61–62. Quotation from Sharp.

48. Greene, *Diary of Carter* 2 : 620, 859–861; Nancy F. Cott, "Eighteenth-Century Family and Social Life revealed in Massachusetts Divorce Records," *Journal of Social History* 10 (Fall 1976): 39.

49. Wright and Tinling, *Diary of William Byrd*, 79; Sharp, *Compleat Midwife's Companion*, 70, alleges that in Great Britain "not one in Twenty" women with their first child even know when their child is due and are surprised by labor.

50. Aristotle (pseud.), *Compleat and Experienc'd Midwife*, 28–30; Morris Braude, *Life Begins: Childbirth in Lore and Literature* (Chicago, 1935), 21–34; Ray B. Browne, *Popular Beliefs and Practices from Alabama*, University of California Publication Folklore Studies, no. 9 (Berkeley, 1958), 8, 10–11; Wayland D. Hand, *Popular Beliefs and Superstitions from North Carolina*, vol. 6, The Frank C. Brown Collection of North Carolina Folklore (Durham, N.C., 1961), 17–23.

51. Cotton Mather, *Diary of Cotton Mather* (New York, 1957), 1 : 163.

52. Mather, *Elizabeth in Her Holy Retirement*, 21–22; Oliver, *A Present for Teeming American Women*, 38.

53. Aristotle (pseud.), *Compleat and Experienc'd Midwife*, 30; Culpeper, *A Directory for Midwives* (London, 1651 edition), 157; Sharp, *Compleat Midwife's Companion*, 113; Spruill, *Women's Life and Work*, 50–51. The General Court of Virginia in 1625 entertained Elizabeth Hamer's complaint that a Dr. Pott had denied her a piece of pork, thereby causing her to miscarry. The judge ruled that Pott's action was not criminal because he did not know that "she had A longing to it." Quotation from Aristotle.

54. Mather, *Ornaments*, 104; Oliver, *A Present for Teeming American Women*, 71.

55. Greene, *Diary of Carter* 2 : 610.

56. Oliver, *A Present for Teeming American Women*, 6.

57. Mather, *Elizabeth in Her Holy Retirement*, 1–2, 6–7; Mather, *Diary* 2 : 618, 700.

58. Oliver, *A Present for Teeming American Women*, 3.

59. Ibid., 118.

60. Calhoun, *Social History of the American Family*, 89.

61. Demos, *Little Commonwealth*, 66, 131–132.

62. David Wallace, ed., *The Life of Henry Laurens* (New York, 1915), 180.

63. Drinker, *Not So Long Ago*, 4, 10, 55–58. On injury during childbirth see Alfred McClintock, ed., *Smellie's Treatise on the Theory and Practice of Midwifery* (London, 1876–1878), 237–239; Willughby, *Observations in Midwifery*, 54, 159. Smellie, in the middle of the eighteenth century, from his own experience judged attempts at repair of tears "impracticable"; once torn, a woman must "continue in that miserable situation." This was the same judgment that Willughby had made the century before.

64. Anne Bradstreet, "Before the Birth of One of her Children," in *Poems of Anne Bradstreet*, ed. Robert Hutchinson (New York, 1969), 45.

65. [Clap], "Memoirs of a College President," 235.

66. Stewart Mitchell, ed., *New Letters of Abigail Adams, 1788–1801* (Boston, 1947), 3–5, 56; Chapman, "Benjamin Colman's Daughters," *New England Quarterly* 26 (1953);

182; Lovell, *Two Quaker Sisters*, 1, 12; Drinker, *Not So Long Ago*, 51–60; Mary Vial Holyoke, diary, *The Holyoke Diaries*, 70, 73, 75, 83, 95, 100, 101, 107; Wallett, "Diary of Parkman," 446–448; Sewall, *Diary* 1 : 11, 40, 110, 166, 222–223, 351, 394, 426; 2 : 49; Ethel Armes, ed., *Nancy Shippen: Her Journal Book* (Philadelphia, 1935), 122–124.

67. James Hobson Aveling, *English Midwives: Their History and Prospects* (1872; reprint London, 1967), 3–4, 7, 10; Edward H. Carter, *The Norwich Subscription Books: A Study of the Subscription Books of the Diocese of Norwich, 1637–1800* (London, 1937), 17–18, 134; Forbes, *The Midwife and the Witch*, 139–145 (see Chapter 10, "Early Regulation of English Midwives").

68. Cutter and Viets, *Short History*, 5–55; Flack, *Eternal Eve*, 218–219; McClintock, *Smellie's Treatise* 2 : 248–250; 3 : 26–27, 298, 317–319; Willughby, *Observations in Midwifery*, 37, 155. Save for midwifery, medical practice in England was divided among three guilds of physicians, surgeons, and apothecaries. Physicians, titled "doctors," and usually possessing university degrees, theoretically as gentlemen did not work with their hands. Surgeons, trained by apprenticeship and rarely holding degrees, dealt with structural emergencies. Apothecaries, also apprenticed, sold medicines. These distinctions disappeared in the rural areas and small towns of England, as well as in colonial America, where medical men, usually without formal training, and indiscriminately called doctors, engaged in general practice. Even after 1765 the Americans who were by strict definition physicians practiced general medicine. Shryock, *Medicine and Society in America*, 2–3, 7, 10.

69. Sharp, *Compleat Midwife's Companion*, xi.

70. *The Midwives Just Petition, or, A Complaint of divers good Gentlewomen of that Faculty* (London, 1643), 1–2; Willughby, *Observations in Midwifery*, 73. Quotations from "Midwives Just Petition."

71. *The Compleat Midwife's Practice, in the Most Weighty and High Concernments of the Birth of Man. by T.C.I.D.M.S.T.B.*, *Practitioners* (London, 1656), 119–124. Quotations from p. 120 of a section entitled "Instructions of a Midwife to Her Daughter" from the book cited above.

72. Aveling, *English Midwives*, 138–144; Clark, *Working Life of Women in the Seventeenth Century*, 265, 269, 270–275; *The Compleat Midwife's Practice*, 119–124; John Memis, *The Midwive's Pocket Companion: or, a Practical Treatise on Midwifery* (London, 1765), v–vii; Sharp, *Compleat Midwife's Companion*, x–xii; Willughby, *Observations in Midwifery*, ix, 73.

73. Aveling, *English Midwives*, 98–101; John Kobler, *The Reluctant Surgeon: A Biography of John Hunter* (New York, 1960), 31; Sharp, *Compleat Midwife's Companion*, Introduction; Willughby, *Observations in Midwifery*, 1–2.

74. Valentine Seaman, *The Midwives Monitor and the Mothers Mirror: Being Three Concluding Lectures of a Course of Instruction of Midwifery* (New York, 1800), viii.

75. Seaman, *Midwives Monitor*, viii. See also Joseph Brevitt, *The Female Medical Repository . . .* (Baltimore, 1810), 6. Quotation from Seamen.

76. Beall, *"Aristotle's Master Piece,"* 209–210; Seaman, *Midwives Monitor*, ix. Beall's article is the best study of the popular manuals of "Aristotle." The *Master Piece*, which was the creation of an English physician, "W.S.," and a succession of hack writers, first appeared in England in 1684. The numerous later editions were the only works on sex and gynecology widely available to eighteenth-century Americans. Quotation from Seaman.

77. Jane B. Donegan, *Women and Men Midwives: Medicine, Morality, and Misogyny in*

Early America (Westport, Conn., 1978), 91–94; "A Law for Regulating Mid Wives Within the City of New York," Minutes of the Common Council of New York, 1716, Appendix I in Claire E. Fox, "Pregnancy, Childbirth and Early Infancy in Anglo-American Culture, 1765–1830" (Ph.D. diss., University of Pennsylvania, 1966), 442–445; "A Law for Regulating Midwives Within the City of New York," *New York Weekly Journal*, June 6, 1738, 241; Richard H. Shryock, *Medical Licensing in America, 1650–1965* (Baltimore, 1967), 3, 16; James J. Walsh, *History of Medicine in New York: Three Centuries of Medical Progress* (New York, 1919), 2 : 22, 25. Quotation is from the 1716 oath.

78. Cutter and Viets, *Short History*, 145, 150; *Maryland Gazette* (Annapolis), Sept. 30, 1747; Francis R. Packard, *History of Medicine in the United States* (New York, 1931), 1 : 52–53; Shryock, *Medicine and Society*, 11–12; J. Whitridge Williams, *A Sketch of the History of Obstetrics in the United States up to 1860* (Baltimore, 1903), 1.

79. Kate Campbell Mead, *A History of Women in Medicine from Earliest Times to the Beginning of the Nineteenth Century* (New York, 1938), 411; Packard, *History of Medicine in the United States* 1 : 44; Herbert Thoms, *Chapters in American Obstetrics*, 2d ed. (Springfield, Ill., 1961), 3.

80. Wyndham B. Blanton, *Medicine in Virginia in the Seventeenth Century* (Richmond, Va., 1930), 166; MS deposition of Sarah Woodward, 1694, Taunton, Massachusetts, bound in Samuel Abbot Green, *History of Medicine in Massachusetts* (Boston, 1881); Packard, *History of Medicine*, 1 : 52; Spruill, *Women's Life and Work*, 272; Thoms, *Chapters in American Obstetrics*, 10.

81. Martha Moore Ballard, diary, in *The History of Augusta: First Settlements and Early Days as a Town, Including the Diary of Mrs. Martha Moore Ballard, 1785–1812*, ed. Charles Eleventon Nash (Augusta, Maine, 1904 [issued 1961]); especially see page 298, where Ballard notes that a doctor copied her records of births and deaths, and page 448, when a man inquires for his birth date; M. D. Learned and C. F. Brede, "An Old German Midwife's Record, Kept by Susanna Muller, of Providence Township, Lancaster County, Pennsylvania, during the years 1791–1815," n.d., Hist. Colls., College of Physicians of Philadelphia.

82. Sewall, *Diary* 1 : 40, 114; Sharp, *Compleat Midwife's Companion*, frontispiece of midwife at christening.

83. Aristotle (pseud.), *Compleat and Experienc'd Midwife*, iii.

84. Broadside of elegy to Mary Broadwell in Francisco Guerra, *American Medical Bibliography, 1693–1783* (New York, 1962), 69.

85. Packard, *History of Medicine*, 1 : 49.

86. Aristotle (pseud.), *Compleat and Experienc'd Midwife*, frontispiece of lying-in; Drinker, *Not So Long Ago*, 51–54, 59; Dow, *Holyoke Diaries*, 70, 73, 75, 81, 83, 95, 101, 107; Wallet, "Diary of Parkman," 446–448; Sewall, *Diary* 5 : 40, 222–223, 394; 6 : 49; Sharp, *Compleat Midwife's Companion*, frontispiece of lying-in; Charles White, *A Treatise on the Management of Pregnant and Lying-in Women* (Worcester, Mass., 1793), 19–20. The itemized bill for her lying-in that an unwed mother submitted to the Middlesex County Massachusetts Court in 1743 suggests what the well-off provided for lying-in and what the poor aspired to have. Mary Cheeney's charges for "entertaining the women" were disallowed as excessive, as were "lhougher [beer] . . . biscakes, rice, chocolate, rum and spirits." The court approved expenditures for "Child Bed Linen; Bringing the midwife and women; midwife fees; oatmeal; spices; nursing; boarding the nurse; fire and candles." Hendrik Hartog, "The Public Law of a County Court; Judicial Government in Eighteenth Century Massachusetts," *American Journal of Legal History* 20 (October 1976):304.

87. John Craig, "The Autobiography of the Reverend John Craig of Tinkling Spring, Virginia," p. 32. MS, the Historical Foundation of Reformed Churches, Montreat, N.C., typescript of Professor Jon Butler, University of Illinois, Chicago Circle. I am indebted to Prof. Butler for the loan of this typescript. Drinker, *Not So Long Ago*, 52; Sewall, *Diary* 5 : 394. Question from Sewall.

88. Aristotle (pseud.), *Compleat and Experienc'd Midwife*, 51, 53; Samuel Bard, *A Compendium of the Theory and Practice of Midwifery*, 5th ed. (New York, 1819), 188; Culpeper, *A Directory for Midwives* (1651), 167, 170–172; Sharp, *Compleat Midwife's Companion*, 125–128, 130; White, *Treatise on Pregnant Women*, 80; Willughby, *Observations in Midwifery*, 4, 11, 13.

89. Aristotle (pseud.), *Compleat and Experienc'd Midwife*, frontispiece, 50–51; Sharp, *Compleat Midwife's Companion*, frontispiece, 115–125; Spruill, *Woman's Life and Work*, 50; White, *Treatise on Pregnant Women*, 20; Willughby, *Observations in Midwifery*, 20.

90. Aristotle (pseud.), *Compleat and Experienc'd Midwife*, 50, 57; Drinker, *Not So Long Ago*, 60; Sewall *Diary* 5 : 40; Sharp, *Compleat Midwife's Companion*, 124, 128; Harold Speert, *Iconographia Gyniatrica: A Pictorial History of Gynecology and Obstetrics* (Philadelphia, 1973), 265–269; Willughby, *Observations in Midwifery*, 19–20.

91. Seaman, *Midwives Monitor*, 90–91.

92. Drinker, *Not So Long Ago*, 59.

93. William Buchan, *Advice to Mothers on the Subject of Their Own Health* (Charleston, S.C., 1807), 28; *The London Practice of Midwifery by an American Practitioner* (Concord, N.H., 1826), 129; Thomas Chalkey James, "Notes from Drs. Osborne's and Clark's Lectures on Midwifery taken by T. C. James, London 1790–1791," MS, Hist. Colls., College of Physicians of Philadelphia.

94. Aristotle (pseud.), *Compleat and Experienc'd Midwife*, 60; Culpeper, *A Directory for Midwives* (1651), 172–181; William Potts Dewees, *A Compendious System of Midwifery, Chiefly Designed to Facilitate the Inquiries of Those Who may be Pursuing This Branch of Study* (Philadelphia, 1826), 212–213; Sharp, *Compleat Midwife's Companion*, 133. Quotations from Aristotle.

95. Drinker, *Not So Long Ago*, 53, 59.

96. Mrs. Eva Jones, ed., "Extracts from the Journal of Miss Sara Eve," *Pennsylvania Magazine of History and Biography* 5 (1881): 195.

97. Aristotle (pseud.), *Compleat and Experienc'd Midwife*, 87–89; Culpeper, *A Directory for Midwives* (1651), 193–195; Sharp, *Compleat Midwife's Companion*, frontispiece of lying-in, 132; McClintock, *Smellie's Treatise* 1 : 380; White, *Treatise on Pregnant Women*, 20.

98. Lyman H. Butterfield et al., eds., *Adams Family Correspondence* (Cambridge, Mass., 1963), 2 : 282, 292; Mitchell, *New Letters of Abigail Adams*, 4–5; Greene, *Diary of Carter 2: : 86; Dow, *Holyoke Diaries*, 49, 56, 58, 62, 63, 65, 67, 73, 77, 78, 82, 95, 100, 107; Sewall, *Diary* 6 : 50–51.

99. Ernest Caulfield, "Infant Feeding in Colonial America," *Journal of Pediatrics* 41 (December 1952):675; Drinker, *Not So Long Ago*, 52–53, 55, 63–64; Sewall, *Diary* 5 : 40–41, 110–111; 6 : 50–51.

100. Sharp, *Compleat Midwife's Companion*, 132. Leviticus 12 : 1–8. When a woman bears a male child she shall be unclean for seven days, and observe thirty-three days of purification; if she bears a female child, she shall be unclean for fourteen days, and observe sixty-six days of purification.

101. Ballard, diary, 327; Sewall, *Diary* 5 : 394; 6 : 51; Sharp, *Compleat Midwife's Companion*, frontispiece of feast; Speert, *Iconographica Gyniatrica*, 150–152, illustrations of puerperal feasts. Quotation from Sewall.

102. Moreau de Saint-Mery, *Voyage Aux Etats-Unis de L'Amerique, 1793–1798*, ed. Stewart Mims (New Haven, 1913), 310.

103. Mitchell, *New Letters of Adams*, 5; Anna Green Winslow, cited by Alice Morse Earle, *Child Life in Colonial Days* (1899; reprint New York, 1967), 17–19; Dow, *Holyoke Diaries*, 49, 56, 58, 63, 65, 67, 73, 77, 78, 82, 95, 100, 107. Quotations from Earle.

104. Cott, "Eighteenth-Century Family Life," 22–24; David H. Flaherty, *Privacy in Colonial New England* (Charlottesville, Va., 1972), 25–112.

105. Alexander, *The History of Women* 1: table of contents, 358.

CHAPTER 2

1. Cecil K. Drinker, *Not So Long Ago: A Chronicle of Medicine and Doctors in Colonial Philadelphia* (New York, 1937), 59–61.

2. Betsy Copping Corner, *William Shippen, Jr., Pioneer in American Medical Education* (Philadelphia, 1951), 103; Irving S. Cutter and Henry R. Viets, *A Short History of Midwifery* (Philadelphia, 1964), 150.

3. Wistar, quoted in Cutter and Viets, *Short History*, 150.

4. *Kite's Philadelphia Directory for 1815* (Philadelphia, 1815), xi–xii; John Paxton, *The Philadelphia Directory and Register for 1819* (Philadelphia, 1819), n.p.; Robert Desilver, *The Philadelphia Directory and Register for 1824* (Philadelphia, 1824), n.p.

5. Walter Channing (John Ware?), *Remarks on the Employment of Females as Practitioners in Midwifery* (Boston, 1820), 1; *Independent Chronicle and the Universal Advertiser* (Boston), Nov. 8, 1781. Quotations from Channing.

6. William Potts Dewees, *A Compendious System of Midwifery, Chiefly Designed to Facilitate the Inquiries of Those Who may be Pursuing This Branch of Study* (Philadelphia, 1826), xiv.

7. Martha Moore Ballard, diary, in *The History of Augusta: First Settlements and Early Days as a Town, Including the Diary of Mrs. Martha Moore Ballard, 1785–1812*, ed. Charles E. Nash (Augusta, Maine, 1904 [issued 1961]), 229–464; William Buchan, *A Compendium of Domestic Midwifery for the Use of Female Practitioners, Being an Appendix to Buchan's Domestic Medicine* (Charleston, S.C., 1815), 3; Channing, *Remarks on the Employment of Females*, 12; Frances E. Kobrin, "The American Midwife Controversy: A Crisis of Professionalization," *Bulletin of the History of Medicine* 40 (1966): 350; M. D. Learned and C.F. Brede, "An Old German Midwife's Record, Kept by Susanna Muller, of Providence Township, Lancaster County, Pennsylvania, during the years 1791–1815," n.d., Hist. Colls., College of Physicians of Philadelphia; Mrs. Joseph Sarber, Memorandum Kept by Mrs. Joseph Sarber, Midwife at the Falls of the Schuylkill from 1814 to 1831, MS, Historical Society of Pennsylvania, Philadelphia.

8. Drinker, *Not So Long Ago*, 51–52; Dewees, *Compendious System of Midwifery*, 303.

9. Charles M. Andrews, *Colonial Folkways: A Chronicle of American Life in the Reign of the Georges* (New Haven, 1919), 147; Corner, *William Shippen*, 1–2; Maurice Bear Gordon, *Aesculapius Comes to the Colonies: The Story of the Early Days of Medicine in the Thirteen Original Colonies* (Ventnor, N.J., 1949), 156–157, 450–465; John Brett Langstaff, *Dr. Bard of Hyde Park, The Famous Physician of Revolutionary Times, The Man Who Saved Washington's Life* (New York, 1942), 57–58; Francis R. Packard, "How London and Edinburgh Influenced Medicine in Philadelphia in the Eighteenth Century," *College of Physicians of Philadelphia, Transactions*, 3d ser., 53 (1931): 167.

10. Gordon, *Aesculapius*, 465; Francis R. Packard, *History of Medicine in the United States*

(New York, 1931), 1 : 181–230; Packard, "How London and Edinburgh Influenced Medicine," 163, 166.

11. John Morgan, *A Discourse Upon the Institution of Medical Schools in America* (1765; reprint Baltimore, 1937), 33.

12. Samuel Bard, *Two Discourses Dealing with Medical Education in Early New York* (1769, 1819; reprint New York, 1921), 1. See also Peter Middleton, *A Medical Discourse or an Historical Inquiry into the Ancient and Present State of Medicine: the Substance of Which Was Delivered at Opening the Medical School in the City of New York* (New York, 1769), 59–64.

13. Bard, *Two Discourses Dealing with Medical Education*, 14–15; Morgan, *Discourse Upon the Institution of Medical Schools*, 14–17; Richard H. Shryock, *The Development of Modern Medicine: An Interpretation of the Social and Scientific Factors Involved* (Philadelphia, 1936), 58–70. Quotation from Bard.

14. Morgan, *Discourse Upon the Institution of Medical Schools*, 23.

15. Josiah Bartlett, M.D., *A Dissertation on the Progress of Medical Science in the Commonwealth of Massachusetts* (Boston, 1810), 5, 10–13; John Redman Coxe, *A Short View of the Importance and Respectability of the Science of Medicine. Read Before the Philadelphia Medical Society . . .* (Philadelphia, 1800), 15–16; Middleton, *A Medical Discourse*, 67.

16. Packard, *History of Medicine* 2 : 1125–1127; J. Whitridge Williams, *A Sketch of the History of Obstetrics in the United States up to 1850* (Baltimore, 1903), 5–7.

17. *Oxford English Dictionary*, s.v. "obstetrics"; Packard, *History of Medicine* 2 : 1125–1126.

18. Cutter and Viets, *Short History*, 68–98. For a detailed discussion of British man midwives and their methods see Jane Donegan, *Women and Men Midwives: Medicine, Morality, and Mysogyny in Early America* (Westport, Conn., 1978), 38–83.

19. Cutter and Viets, *Short History*, 4–26; Isaac Harvey Flack (pseud. Harvey Graham), *Eternal Eve* (London, 1950), 218.

20. Cutter and Viets, *Short History*, 44–59.

21. Ibid., 26–28, 182.

22. Ibid., 44–59; John Glaister, *Dr. William Smellie and His Contemporaries* (Glasgow, 1894), 170, 174, 178–179, 187; Alfred McClintock, ed., *Smellie's Treatise on the Theory and Practice of Midwifery* (London, 1876–1878), 2 : 250–251, 339.

23. McClintock, ed., *Smellie's Treatise* 1 : 219, 240–241; William Smellie, *Anatomical Tables with Explanations, and an abridgement of the practice of midwifery . . .* (Edinburgh, 1787); Herbert Spencer, *The History of British Midwifery from 1650 to 1800* (London, 1927), 48–50.

24. Cutter and Viets, *Short History*, 35–36; John Kobler, *The Reluctant Surgeon: A Biography of John Hunter* (New York, 1960), 82–83; Spencer, *History of British Midwifery*, 69–71.

25. Corner, *William Shippen*, 53; McClintock, *Smellie's Treatise* 3 : 26–27, 298, 317–318; Spencer, *History of British Midwifery*, Appendix II, 179–182, "British Lying-in Institutions and Their Staffs." All the eighteenth-century physicians after Smellie who contributed significantly to the development of obstetrics by their teaching and published research were on the staffs of lying-in hospitals.

26. McClintock, *Smellie's Treatise* 1 : 78.

27. Charles White, *A Treatise on the Management of Pregnant and Lying-in Women* (Worcester, Mass., 1793), 70–71.

28. Thomas Dashiell Jones, *An Essay on the Importance of the Obstetrick Art; Submitted to the Examination of Charles Alexander Warfield, M.D., President of the Medical Faculty of the College of Medicine of Maryland* (Baltimore, 1812), 5, 11, 21, 23.

29. William Potts Dewees, *Essays on Various Subjects Connected with Midwifery* (Philadelphia, 1823), 25, 33; Thomas Denman, *An Introduction to the Practice of Midwifery* (New York, 1802), 1 : 47; Jones, *Essay on Obstetrick Art*, 8, 17–19; Valentine Seaman, *The Midwives Monitor and the Mothers Mirror: Being Three Concluding Lectures of a Course of Instruction of Midwifery* (New York, 1800), x; White, *Treatise on Pregnant Women*, 79. Quotation from Jones.

30. Carl Bridenbaugh, *Cities in Revolt: Urban Life in America, 1743–1776* (1955; reprint New York, 1971), 216–217; U.S. Department of the Interior, Bureau of the Census, "Population of Cities Having 25,000 Inhabitants or More in 1900, at Each Census: 1790–1900," *Twelfth Census of the United States, Taken in the Year 1900, Population, Part I* (Washington, D.C., 1901), 430–433.

31. Boston Medical Association, *Rules and Regulations of the Boston Medical Association* (Boston, 1806), 4–5. The minimum fee escalated to $15/day case, $20/night by 1819. Boston Medical Association, *Rules and Regulations* (1819 edition).

32. Channing, *Remarks on the Employment of Females*, 19; Edward Warren, *The Life of John Collins Warren, M.D., Compiled Chiefly from His Autobiography and Journals* (Boston, 1860), 1 : 219.

33. Dewees, *Compendious System of Midwifery* (Philadelphia, 1824), 307.

34. Ibid. (Philadelphia, 1826 edition), xiv.

35. Drinker, *Not So Long Ago*, 51, 54–56, 59.

36. Dewees, *Compendious System of Midwifery* (Philadelphia, 1824 edition), 307; Drinker, *Not So Long Ago*, 60.

37. Samuel Bard, *A Compendium of the Theory and Practice of Midwifery*, 5th ed. (New York, 1819), v, 176, 289; Dewees, *Compendious System of Midwifery* (Philadelphia, 1826 edition), xv.

38. Bard, *A Compendium of the Theory and Practice of Midwifery*, iv–v, 289.

39. Dewees, *Compendious System of Midwifery* (Philadelphia, 1826 edition), 302–303.

40. Quotation from Bard, *A Compendium of the Theory and Practice of Midwifery*, viii. Other general statements of the frequency of forceps use appear in Joseph Brevitt, *The Female Medical Repository* . . . (Baltimore, 1810), 149–155, and Warren, *The Life of John Collins Warren*, I, 219–220. Brevitt claims to have delivered "at least 1,000" children without ever using instruments. Warren wrote that he "occasionally" used forceps in the early years of his practice but did so for the last time in 1818; he practiced midwifery for about ten years after that.

41. Denman, *Introduction to Midwifery*, 235.

42. Jones, *Essay on Obstetrick Art*, 23.

43. John R. B. Rodgers, "Presidential Address on Puerperal Fever," *Transactions of the Medical Society of the State of New York* (1815), 11–12.

44. Dewees, *Compendious System of Midwifery* (Philadelphia, 1826 edition), 18.

45. Jones, *Essay on Obstetrick Art*, 8.

46. Peter Miller, *An Essay on the Means of Lessening the Pains of Parturition* (Philadelphia, 1804), 340.

47. Dewees, *Essays on Various Subjects Connected with Midwifery*, 24.

48. Ibid., 25; Miller, *Essay on Lessening the Pains*, 343–348; M. Pierce Rucker, "An Eighteenth Century Method of Pain Relief in Obstetrics," *Journal of the History of Medicine* 5 (Winter 1950): 101–105. One method of pain relief advocated by Miller and used by other physicians as well as copious bloodletting, which by producing relaxation actually did make childbirth more comfortable (ibid., 105.) Quotation from Dewees.

49. David Humphreys Storer, "Lectures on Midwifery. By Walter Channing. Taken at the Medical Colleges, Boston, 1824 and 1825," MS, Countway Collection, Harvard Medical School Library.

50. Brevitt, *Female Medical Repository*, 132–134.

51. Channing, *Remarks on the Employment of Females*, 6–12; Jones, *Essay on Obstetrick Art*, 20; Joseph F. Kett, *The Formation of The American Medical Profession: The Role of Institutions, 1780–1860* (New Haven, 1968), 10–30.

52. James Hobson Aveling, *English Midwives: Their History and Prospects* (1872; reprint London, 1967), 137–144; Glaister, *Dr. William Smellie*, 32–36; John Leake, *A Lecture Introductory to the Theory and Practice of Midwifery* (London, 1773), 31–32; McClintock, ed., *Smellie's Treatise* 1 : 431–432; Spencer, *History of British Midwifery*, 179–181. Quotations from Smellie in the McClintock edition.

53. Cutter and Viets, *Short History*, 28; McClintock, *Smellie's Treatise* 1 : 431–432.

54. Corner, *William Shippen*, 104–105; *Pennsylvania Gazette* (Philadelphia), Jan. 31, 1765; James Thacher, *American Medical Biography* (1828; reprint New York, 1967), 2 : 86. Quotations from Shippen in Corner.

55. Williams, *Sketch of the History of Obstetrics*, 13; Seaman, *Midwives Monitor*, iii–vii. (See note 29, above.)

56. Bard, *Compendium of Theory and Practice of Midwifery*, iv, 289; Brevitt, *Female Medical Repository*, 149–155; Buchan, *Compendium of Domestic Midwifery;* Samuel Jennings, *Married Lady's Companion or Poor Man's Friend* . . . (New York, 1808), 135; Seaman, *Midwives Monitor*, 31–32. All these works were directed entirely or in part to midwives.

57. Thomas Ewell, *Letters to Ladies, Detailing Important Information Concerning Themselves and Infants* (Philadelphia, 1817), vii–viii.

58. Warren, *The Life of John Collins Warren*, 1 : 220; 2 : 276.

59. Channing, *Remarks on the Employment of Females as Practitioners in Midwifery*, 4, 19–20.

60. Ibid., 4, 6–10.

61. Ibid., 4–5.

62. Bard, *Compendium of Theory and Practice of Midwifery*, 188; Dewees, *Compendious System of Midwifery* (Philadelphia, 1826 edition), 190, 203, 212–213.

63. William Baker, Jr., *Cautions to Pregnant and Lying-in Women; Together with Some Hints on Nursing Young Children* (Washington, D.C., 1810), 2.

64. *Essex Gazette* (Salem, Mass.), July 14–21, 1772; *New York Gazette*, July 4, 1768; *Virginia Gazette* (Purdie and Dixon), Nov. 28, 1771, and Dec. 16, 1773. See also Richard H. Shryock, *Medicine in America: Historical Essays* (Baltimore, 1966), 181–182.

65. *New York Gazette*, June 3, 1771.

66. Ballard, diary, in *The History of Augusta*, 243, 244, 251, 271, 273, 286, 290, 298, 299, 309, 318, 326, 327, 336, 338, 345, 361, 373, 374, 377, 379, 386, 390, 400, 442, 451, 459, 463, 464.

67. Ibid., 386, 390. For a more general discussion of competition between physicians and midwives see Donegan, *Women and Men Midwives*, 120–121.

68. Aveling, *English Midwives*, 137–144, 153–159; Cutter and Viets, *Short History*, 43; Glaister, *William Smellie*, 32–36.

69. Dewees, *Compendious System of Midwifery* (Philadelphia, 1826 edition), xv.

70. Channing, *Remarks on Employment of Females*, 16, 17.

71. Ewell, *Letters to Ladies*, 27; Dewees, *Compendious System of Midwifery* (Philadelphia, 1826 edition), 135–136. Dewees was unable to tell his students whether sores always

encrusted the vulva of women suffering from severe vaginal puritis, though he thought it "probable." He had treated nine cases in five years, but he had only "two opportunities of examining the parts."

72. Jones, *Essay on Obstetrick Art*, 11.

73. Seaman, *Midwives Monitor*, iv.

74. *Virginia Gazette* (Purdie and Dixon), Oct. 1, 1772; reprinted in *New-London Gazette* (Conn.), Jan. 29, 1773. The New London editor noted that a "J. C." of Mansfield had sent him a clipping of the article, saying that "by inserting the following you will doubtless oblige many of your constant readers."

75. Elizabeth Nihill, *A Treatise on the Art of Midwifery, Setting Forth Various Abuses Therein. Especially as to the Practice With Instruments* (London, 1760), and S. W. Forbes, *Man-Midwifery Dissected* (London, 1793), are outstanding examples of arguments made about the supposed immorality of man midwives. Donegan discusses the opposition to man midwives at some length in *Women and Men Midwives*, 164–196.

76. Ewell, *Letters to Ladies*, 27.

77. Dewees, *Compendious System of Midwifery* (Philadelphia, 1826 edition), 189; Daniel B. Smith, "Notes on Lectures of Thomas Chalkey James and William Potts Dewees, University of Pennsylvania, 1826," MS, Hist. Colls., College of Physicians of Philadelphia.

78. *The London Practice of Midwifery by an American Practitioner* (Concord, N.H., 1826), 109.

79. Bard, *Compendium of Theory and Practice of Midwifery*, 181; lecture notes from lectures of William Shippen, Jr., University of Pennslyvania, n.d., MS, Hist. Colls., College of Physicians of Philadelphia.

80. Bard, *Compendium of Theory and Practice of Midwifery*, 181; Dewees, *Compendious System of Midwifery* (Philadelphia, 1826 edition), 189–190; *London Practice of Midwifery*, 108–109; Storer, "Notes on Channing's Lectures on Midwifery," MS, Countway Collection, Harvard Medical School Library.

81. Thomas Denman, *The Obstetrical Remembrancer, or Denman's Aphorisms on Natural and Difficult Parturition* (New York, 1848; orig. U.S. pub., 1803), 46.

82. *London Practice of Midwifery*, 129.

83. Dewees, *Compendious System of Midwifery* (Philadelphia, 1826 edition), 190; *London Practice of Midwifery*, 129–130; Storer, "Notes on Channing's Lectures on Midwifery," MS, Countway Collection, Harvard Medical School Library.

84. Thomas Chalkey James, "Notes from Drs. Osborne's and Clark's Lectures on Midwifery taken by T. C. James, London, 1790–91"; MS, Hist. Colls., College of Physicians of Philadelphia; Notes on Shippen lectures, Hist. Colls., College of Physicians of Philadelphia; *London Practice of Midwifery*, 127.

85. Ibid.

86. Storer, "Notes on Channing's Lectures on Midwifery."

87. Dewees, *Compendious System of Midwifery*, (Philadelphia, 1826 edition), 190.

88. Bard, *Compendium of Theory and Practice of Midwifery*, 190–191, Seaman, *Midwives Monitor*, ix.

89. Bard, *Compendium of Theory and Practice of Midwifery*, 220; Seaman, *Midwives Monitor*, ix.

90. Dewees, *Compendious System of Midwifery* (Philadelphia, 1826 edition), 313.

91. Kobler, *Reluctant Surgeon*, 32; *London Practice of Midwifery*, 132–133.

92. For a thoughtful discussion of the conflict between the increasing emphasis on

female modesty in the late eighteenth and early nineteenth centuries, and efforts to make midwifery the exclusive province of men, see Donegan, *Women and Men Midwives*, 149–157.

93. Thomas Jefferson to Mary Jefferson Eppes, December 26, 1803, in *The Domestic Life of Thomas Jefferson, Compiled from Family Letters and Reminiscences by his Great Granddaughter* ed. Sarah N. Randolph (Cambridge, Mass., 1939), 252–253.

CHAPTER 3

1. Charlotte Perkins Gilman, *Women and Economics, A Study of the Economic Relation Between Men and Women as a Factor in Social Evolution*, ed. Carl Degler (1898; reprint New York, 1966), 174.

2. Ibid., 176; G. F. Root, "Just Before the Battle, Mother," in *Fireside Book of Favorite American Songs*, ed. Margaret Bradford Boni (New York, 1952), 153–155.

3. Gilman, *Women and Economics*, 171. Two general surveys that describe the general development and characteristics of modern family life in Western Europe and America are: Patricia Branca, *Women in Europe Since 1750* (London, 1978), and Edward Shorter, *The Making of the Modern Family* (New York, 1975), especially Chapter 5, "Mothers and Infants."

4. Elizabeth Anthony Dexter, *Colonial Women of Affairs: Women in Business and the Professions in America Before 1776*, 2d ed. (Boston, 1931), 185, 189–192. See variations on this argument in: Mary Ryan, *Womanhood in America from Colonial Times to the Present* (New York, 1975); Page Smith, *Daughters of the Promised Land: Women in American History* (Boston, 1970); and Ann D. Gordon and Mary Jo Buhle, "Sex and Class in Colonial and Nineteenth Century America," and Alice Kessler Harris, "Women, Work and the Social Order," both in *Liberating Women's History*, ed. Berenice A. Carroll (Urbana, Ill., 1976).

5. John Demos, *A Little Commonwealth: Family Life in Plymouth Colony* (New York, 1970), 84–91; Richard B. Morris, *Studies in the History of American Law, with Special Reference to the Seventeenth and Eighteenth Centuries*, 2d ed. (Philadelphia, 1959), 126–200; Roger Thompson, *Women in Stuart England and America: A Comparative Study* (London, 1974), 161–181.

6. Marylynn Salmon, "Equality or Submission? Femme Covert Status in Early Pennsylvania," in *Women of America: A History*, ed. Carol Ruth Berkin and Mary Beth Norton (Boston, 1979), 92–113. See also Lyle Koehler, *A Search for Power: The "Weaker Sex" in Seventeenth Century New England* (Urbana, Ill., 1980), 49–52, for a discussion of women's legal status in Puritan New England.

7. George Saville, Lord Halifax, *The Lady's New-Year's Gift or: Advice to a Daughter* (1700; reprint Stamford, Conn., 1934), 16, 47. Two histories survey the didactic literature for women in the colonies: Mary Sumner Benson, *Women in Eighteenth Century America: A Study of Opinion and Social Usage* (1935; reprint Chapel Hill, N.C., 1972), and Julia Cherry Spruill, *Women's Life and Work in the Southern Colonies* (1938; reprint Chapel Hill, N.C., 1972), Chapter 10, "The Lady's Library."

8. Cotton Mather, *Ornaments for the Daughters of Zion, or the Character and Happiness of a Woman*, 3d ed. (Boston, 1741), 89. See discussions of this point in: Benson, *Women in Eighteenth Century America*, 33; Demos, *Little Commonwealth*, 82–84; William and Malleville Haller, "The Puritan Art of Love," *Huntington Library Quarterly* 5 (January 1942): 235–272; Edmund S. Morgan, *The Puritan Family: Religion and Domestic Relations in Sev-

enteenth Century New England, rev. ed. (New York, 1966), 41–48; Benjamin Wadsworth, *The Well-Ordered Family: or, Relative Duties* (Boston, 1712), 29, 35.

9. Mather, *Ornaments*, 95.

10. Demos, *Little Commonwealth*, 84–95; Dexter, *Colonial Women of Affairs;* W. and M. Haller, "Puritan Art of Love," 249; Spruill, *Women's Life and Work*, 255–313; Thompson, *Women in Stuart England and America*.

11. *Pennsylvania Packet*, Sept. 23, 1780, advertisement cited in Alice Morse Earle, *Home Life in Colonial Days* (1898; reprint New York, 1966), 252. The first five chapters of Mary Beth Norton, *Liberty's Daughters: The Revolutionary Experience of American Women, 1750– 1800* (Boston, 1980), contain the best available description of women's household work and their feelings about it in the late eighteenth century. Earle's *Home Life* provides detailed descriptions of the tasks of colonial housewifery. See also Laurel Thatcher Ulrich, *Good Wives: Image and Reality in the Lives of Women in Northern New England, 1650– 1750* (New York, 1982), 15–30, for a discussion of varieties of household tasks among northern New England women.

12. Mary Cooper, diary, cited in Norton, *Liberty's Daughters*, 11.

13. Edith Abbott, *Women in Industry: A Study in American Economic History* (New York, 1910), 10–34; Earle, *Home Life in Colonial Days*, 166–251; Norton, *Liberty's Daughters*, 15–20.

14. Benjamin Franklin, *The Autobiography of Benjamin Franklin*, ed. Henry Steele Commager (New York, 1950), 90.

15. Alice Clark, *Working Life of Women in the Seventeenth Century* (1919; reprint New York, 1968), 150–235.

16. Antenuptial agreement of Elizabeth Murray Smith and Ralph Inman, September 24, 1771, appended to Mary Beth Norton, "A Cherished Spirit of Independence: The Life of an Eighteenth Century Boston Businesswoman," in Berkin and Norton, *Women of America*, 61–64.

17. Mary Beth Norton, "Eighteenth Century American Women in Peace and War: The Case of the Loyalists," *William and Mary Quarterly*, 3d ser., 33 (July 1976) : 388– 394.

18. Ulrich, *Good Wives*, 157.

19. John Abbott, *The Mother at Home; or The Principles of Maternal Duty, Familiarly Illustrated* (New York, 1833), 10; An American Matron, *The Maternal Physician, A Treatise on the Nurture and Management of Infants . . .* (New York, 1811), dedication page.

20. Halifax, *The Lady's New-Year's Gift*, 43–51; Cotton Mather, *A Family Well Ordered, or an Essay to render Parents and Children Happy in one another . . .* (Boston, 1699), 26, 36–37; Spruill, *Women's Life and Work*, 55; Wadsworth, *The Well-Ordered Family* (Boston, 1712), 46.

21. Grace Abbott, *The Child and the State* (Chicago, 1938), 1 : 5–8; Benson, *Women in Eighteenth Century America*, 239–240; William Blackstone, *Commentaries on the Laws of England*, ed. William Carey Jones (San Francisco, 1916), 1 : 647–648; Helen I. Clarke, *Social Legislation*, 2nd ed. (New York, 1957), 216–225; Spruill, *Women's Life and Work*, 344–346.

22. Philip J. Greven, Jr., *Four Generations: Population, Land, and Family in Colonial Andover, Massachusetts* (Ithaca, N.Y., 1970), 74–99; Daniel Scott Smith, "Parental Power and Marriage Patterns: An Analysis of Historical Trends: Hingham, Massachusetts," in *The American Family in Social-Historical Perspective*, ed. Michael Gordon, 2d ed. (New York, 1978), 87–100; Spruill, *Women's Life and Work*, 345–346; Laurence Stone, "The

Rise of the Nuclear Family in Early Modern England: The Patriarchal Stage," in *The Family in History*, ed. Charles Rosenberg (Philadelphia, 1975), 35–36.

23. Mather, *A Family Well Ordered*, 2–8; Morgan, *The Puritan Family*, 12–28; Stone, "Rise of the Nuclear Family," 34–36, 44–57; Wadsworth, *The Well-Ordered Family*, 1.

24. Clayton H. Chapman, "Benjamin Colman's Daughters," *New England Quarterly* 26 (1953) : 171–174; Christopher Hill, *Society and Puritanism in Pre-Revolutionary England* (New York, 1964), 443–481; Cotton Mather, *Diary of Cotton Mather* (New York, 1957), 2 : 25, 144, 149; Morgan, *The Puritan Family*, 29–32; Stone, "Rise of the Nuclear Family," 29–32.

25. Journal of Esther Burr, 1754, cited in Philip J. Greven, Jr., *The Protestant Temperament: Patterns of Child-Rearing, Religious Experience, and the Self in Early America* (New York, 1977), 35. The term "slaves of Divels" appears in Mather, *A Family Well Ordered*, 12. The best survey of the religious meanings of American Puritan childrearing practices appears in Greven, *The Protestant Temperament*, in a chapter on what he calls evangelical childrearing (pp. 28–55). Other reviews of the material appear in Morgan, *The Puritan Family*, 75–78; David E. Stannard, "Death and the Puritan Child," in *Death in America*, ed. David E. Stannard (Philadelphia, 1975), 19–21.

26. Mather, *A Family Well Ordered*, 37.

27. Halifax, *The Lady's New-Year's Gift*, 51; John Locke, *Some Thoughts Concerning Education* (1692; reprint Cambridge, Mass., 1913), lxi–lxiii, 28, 78–80; Spruill, *Women's Life and Work*, 55; Wadsworth, *The Well-Ordered Family*, 45–46.

28. Benjamin Colman, *Some of the Honours that Religion Does Unto the Fruitful Mothers in Israel . . .* (Boston, 1715), 12, 14, 17; Mather, *Ornaments*, 109; Wadsworth, *The Well-Ordered Family*, 76.

29. Halifax, *The Lady's New-Year's Gift*, 48.

30. Anne Bradstreet, *Poems of Anne Bradstreet*, ed. Robert Hutchinson (New York, 1969); see "In reference to her Children," June 1656, pp. 47–49. Eliza Lucas Pinckney to Miss Bartlett, 1745, printed in Harriott Harry Ravenel, *Eliza Pinckney* (New York, 1896), 109.

31. Thomas Foxcroft, *A Sermon Preach'd at Cambridge, After the Funeral of Mrs. Elizabeth Foxcroft . . .* (Boston, 1721), 30; Cotton Mather, *Maternal Consolations, An Essay on the Consolations of God . . .* (Boston, 1714), 18–19; Greven, *The Protestant Temperament*, pp. 22–24, reviews the recollections of other Puritans who associated their mothers with love.

32. Mather, *Ornaments*, 6.

33. Foxcroft, *A Sermon Preach'd at Cambridge*, 7–8, 13–14, 33, 38; Mather, *Maternal Consolations*, 44.

34. "Ambivalence" is the exact word that John Wulzer uses to title his survey of eighteenth-century childrearing: John Wulzer, "A Period of Ambivalence: Eighteenth-Century American Childhood," in *The History of Childhood*, ed. Lloyd De Mause (New York, 1975), 351–382.

35. Samuel Willard, cited in David E. Stannard, *The Puritan Way of Death: A Study in Religion, Culture and Social Change* (New York, 1977), 52; see also Greven's survey of Puritan definitions of children's value in *The Protestant Temperament*, 28–31.

36. Greven, *The Protestant Temperament*, 32–43; Stannard, *Puritan Way of Death*, 50.

37. John Earle, 1628, cited in Stannard, *Puritan Way of Death*, 48.

38. Greven, *The Protestant Temperament*, esp. pp. 164–165, 159–170, 276–281.

39. Sally Logan Fisher, diary, August 7, 1779, cited in Norton, *Liberty's Daughters*,

96. See also Norton's summary of women's thoughts on the importance of discipline, ibid., 95–97; and Greven, *The Protestant Temperament*, 159–191, especially his discussion of Abigail Adams, Mercy Otis Warren, and the Philadelphia Quakers.

40. Nancy Cott, "Eighteenth-Century Family and Social Life Revealed in Massachusetts Divorce Records," *Journal of Social History* 10 (Fall 1976) : 28–30. Cott bases her conclusions on 220 petitions for divorce or separation presented to the court between 1692 and 1786.

41. Norton, *Liberty's Daughters*, 85.

42. H. L. Mencken, *The American Language: An Inquiry into the Development of English in the United States, Supplement II* (New York, 1948), 474; Norton, *Liberty's Daughters*, 85–87; Lawrence Stone, *The Family, Sex and Marriage in England 1500–1800* (New York, 1977), 409; Daniel Scott Smith, "Child-Naming Patterns and Family Structure Change: Hingham, Massachusetts, 1640–1880," Newberry Library Papers in Family and Community History, no. 76, January 1977. Female children were also commonly named after mothers and other relatives; see Ulrich, *Good Wives*, 150–152.

43. James Axtell, *The School Upon A Hill: Education and Society in Colonial New England* (New Haven, 1974), 85–86; William Cadogan, *An Essay Upon Nursing and the Management of Children from Their Birth to Three Years of Age*, 10th ed. (Boston, 1772), 12; Joseph Illick, "Child-Rearing in Seventeenth-Century England and America," in *The History of Childhood*, ed. Lloyd De Mause (New York, 1975), 307, 325; John Rendle-Short, "Infant Management in the Eighteenth Century with a Special Reference to the Work of William Cadogan," *Bulletin of the History of Medicine* 34 (March 1960) : 100–108; Stone, *The Family, Sex and Marriage*, 161–162; Wadsworth, *The Well-Ordered Family*, 45; Mary Watkins, *Maternal Solicitude, or, Lady's Manual . . .* (New York, 1809), 12–15.

44. Ernest Caulfield, "Infant Feeding in Colonial America," *Journal of Pediatrics* 41 (December 1952) : 673–687; Mather, *Ornaments*, 105; Samuel Sewall, *Diary of Samuel Sewall*, Massachusetts Historical Society Collections, 5th Ser., 5 vols. (1878–1882), 5 : 40, 288; Rendle-Short, "Infant Management," 112–115; Stone, *The Family, Sex and Marriage*, 426–432; Wadsworth, *The Well-Ordered Family*, 46.

45. Cecil K. Drinker, *Not So Long Ago: A Chronicle of Medicine and Docters in Colonial Philadelphia* (New York, 1937), 63–64; Caulfield, "Infant Feeding," 677–681; Spruill, *Women's Life and Work*, 55–57; John Walzer, "A Period of Ambivalence: Eighteenth Century American Childhood," in *The History of Childhood*, ed. Lloyd De Mause (New York, 1975), 353–355.

46. Margaret Mead and Miles Newton, "Cultural Patterning of Prenatal Behavior," in *Childbearing—Its Social and Psycological Aspects*, ed. Stephen Richardson and Alan F. Guttmacher (Baltimore, 1967), 182–187; Spruill, *Women's Life and Work*, 56. For a review of current literature on the psychology of maternal breast-feeding see Susan (Contratto) Weisskopf, "Review Essay: Maternal Sexuality and Asexual Motherhood," *Signs* 5 (Summer 1980) : 778, 780.

47. Demos, *Little Commonwealth*, 69; Greven, *The Protestant Temperament*, 152–156.

48. Philip J. Greven, Jr., "The Average Size of Families and Households in the Province of Massachusetts in 1764 and in the United States in 1790: An Overview," in *The Household and Family in Past Time*, ed. Peter Laslett and Richard Wall (Cambridge, England 1972), 548–551.

49. Greven, *The Protestant Temperament*, 274–276.

50. Robert H. Bremner, ed., *Children and Youth in America: A Documentary History, Volume I: 1600–1865* (Cambridge, Mass., 1970), 103–122, especially 103–105; Demos,

Little Commonwealth, 75–78; Morgan, *The Puritan Family*, 74–78; Spruill, *Women's Life and Work*, 57–59. Although the law defined servitude and apprenticeship as separate institutions, apprenticeship was in fact often really a specialized form of servitude. The main distinction between apprenticeship and servitude was the master's obligation to teach the apprentice a specific trade; servants were bound by indenture to serve a number of years, without specification of the type of labor. See Bremner, *Children and Youth in America* 1 : 104.

51. Edith Abbott, "A Study of the Early History of Child Labor in America," *American Journal of Sociology* 14 (July 1908) : 15–21; Bremner, *Children and Youth in America* 1 : 103–105.

52. Demos, *Little Commonwealth*, 74–75; Morgan, *The Puritan Family*, 75–78.

53. Demos, *Little Commonwealth*, 74–75.

54. Alice Morse Earle, *Child Life in Colonial Days* (1899; reprint New York, 1967), vii.

55. Philippe Ariès, *Centuries of Childhood: A Social History of Family Life*, trans. Robert Baldick (New York, 1962), 128–129; Stannard, "Death and the Puritan Child," 11–15.

CHAPTER 4

1. John Locke, *Some Thoughts Concerning Education*, Introduction and Notes by R. H. Quick (1692; reprint Cambridge, Mass., 1913), lxiii, 4–5; David Ramsay, *Memoirs of the Life of Martha Laurens Ramsay . . .* (Philadelphia, 1811), 39; Harriott Harry Ravenel, *Eliza Pinckney* (New York, 1896), 113.

2. [John Hill], *On the Education and Management of Children, . . . by the Honourable Julianna-Susannah Seymour* (London, 1754); Abigail Adams to Mercy Otis Warren, July 16, 1773, in *Adams Family Correspondence*, ed. Lyman H. Butterfield et al. (Cambridge, Mass., 1963, 1973), 1 : 84.

3. The best surveys of early American (1785–1860) childrearing literature are: Ruth Block, "American Feminine Ideals in Transition: The Rise of the Moral Mother, 1785–1815," *Feminist Studies* 4 (June 1978): 101–126; Anne L. Kuhn, *The Mother's Role in Childhood Education: New England Concepts, 1830–1860* (New Haven, 1947); and Nancy F. Cott, *The Bonds of Womanhood: "Woman's Sphere" in New England, 1780–1835* (New Haven, 1977), which analyzes ministerial sermons and maternal responsibility and appends a bibliography of sermons. See also bibliography in Bernard Wishy, *The Child and the Republic: The Dawn of Modern American Child Nurture* (Philadelphia, 1968). Periodical literature for women is surveyed in: Bertha M. Stearns, "Early New England Magazines for Ladies," *New England Quarterly* 11 (July 1929) : 420–457, and Stearns, "New England Magazines for Ladies," *New England Quarterly* 3 (October 1930) : 627–656.

4. David A. Strong, "Maternal Responsibility," *Mother's Assistant* 21 (1851) : 97–101.

5. Examples of work in which generalizations about behavior are heavily based on prescriptive on literature and fiction, include Wishy, *The Child and the Republic: The Dawn of Modern American Child Nurture* (Philadephia, 1968), William E. Bridges, "Family Patterns and Social Values in America, 1825–75," *American Quarterly* (1965) : 3–11; Kirk Jeffrey, Jr., "Family History: The Middle-Class American Family in the Urban Context, 1830–1870" (Ph.D. diss., Stanford University, 1971); Barbara Welter, "The Cult of True Womanhood, 1820–1860," in *Dimity Convictions: The American Woman in the Nineteenth Century* (Athens, Ohio, 1976), 21–41.

6. Carl N. Degler, "What Ought to Be and What Was: Women's Sexuality in the Nineteenth Century," *American Historical Review* 79 (December 1974) : 1467–1490, crit-

icizes historians of Victorian sexuality for taking prescriptive medical literature as descriptive. Jay Mechling explains these and other cautions on using didactic literature in "Advice to Historians on Advice to Mothers," *Journal of Social History* 9 (Fall 1975) : 44–63. See also "Comment" on this article and "Author's Response," *Journal of Social History* 10 (Fall 1976) : 124–128.

7. John Abbott, *The Mother at Home; or The Principles of Maternal Duty Familiarly Illustrated* (New York, 1833), 10.

8. Daniel Chaplin, *A Discourse delivered before The Charitable Female Society in Groton, October 19, 1814* (Andover, Mass., 1814), 10.

9. Margaret Coxe, *Claims of the Country on American Females* (Columbus, Ohio, 1842), 2 : 38.

10. W. R. Wallace, "John O'Londen's Treasure Trove," (?–1881) cited in *The Penguin Dictionary of Quotations*, ed. John and M. J. Cohen (Harmmondsworth, England, 1960), 408.

11. Anne Kuhn considers in detail the range of advice offered on all three areas of childrearing in her history, *The Mother's Role in Childhood Education*. Anyone interested in an exhaustive analysis of mid-nineteenth-century didactic literature for mothers should consult her work.

12. Lydia N. Sigourney, *Letters to Mothers* (Hartford, Conn., 1838), 32, 114; Lydia Child, *The Mother's Book* 2d ed. (Boston, 1831), 4.

13. (A Physician of New York), author of "Supplementary Chapter," in Louisa M. Barwell, *Infant Treatment: With Directions to Mothers for Self-Management Before, During, and After Pregnancy. Addressed to Mothers and Nurses . . .* (first American edition: New York, 1844), 120–125. Statistics showed an average mortality rate of 43% under five years during nine years before he wrote. He found the ratio higher in New York (50% in 1840), Philadelphia (51% in 1839), and in southern cities of Charleston, Savannah, Mobile, New Orleans "even greater." He found an increase of mortality in New York City (1810, 32%; 1820, 38%; 1830, 44% under five) and Boston (1810–20, 27%; 1831–39, 43%). pp. 120–121.

14. Kuhn makes this argument in *The Mother's Role in Childhood Education*, 6–7, and Chapter 6, "Guardian of the Temple of the Immortal Soul," 120–148.

15. William Cadogan, *An Essay Upon Nursing and the Management of Children from Their Birth to Three Years of Age*, 10th ed. (Boston, 1772), 34.

16. William Baker, Jr., M.D., *Cautions to Pregnant and Lying-in Women; Together With Some Hints on Nursing Young Children* (Washington, D.C., 1810), 9–10; Cadogan, *An Essay Upon Nursing*, 19–20; Willaim Mathews Treland, *Advice to Mothers, on the Management of Infants . . .* (New York, 1820), 5, 12. Quotation from Baker.

17. (A Physician of New York), *Infant Treatment*, 122–125, 129; Cadogan, *An Essay Upon Nursing*, 22–23; J. C. Drummond and Anne Wilbraham, *The Englishman's Food: A History of Five Centuries of English Diet*, rev. ed. (London, 1958) 244–249; Kuhn, *The Mother's Role in Childhood Education*, 136–139; John Rendle-Short, "Infant Management in the Eighteenth Century with a special Reference to the Work of William Cadogan," *Bulletin of the History of Medicine* 34 (March 1960) : 112–117.

18. William Alcott, *The Young Mother, or Management of Children in Regard to Health* 2d ed. (Boston, 1836), 115–139; (A Physician of New York), *Infant Treatment*, 128–131; Cadogan, *An Essay Upon Nursing*, 22–24; Treland, *Advice to Mothers*, 5–7; Kuhn, *The Mother's Role in Childhood Education*, 139–141; Rendle-Short, "Infant Management," 117–120; Hugh Smith, M.D., *The Female Monitor, Consisting of a Series of Letters to Married*

Women on the Nursing and Management of Children . . . (Wilmington, Del. 1801), ix, 94–95; Robert Sunley. "Early Nineteenth-Century American Literature on Child Rearing," in *Childhood in Contemporary Cultures*, ed. Margaret Mead and Martha Wolfenstein (Chicago, 1954), 153–155.

19. Mary Watkins, *Maternal Solicitude, or, Lady's Manual: Comprising a Brief View of the happy advantages resulting from an early attention to secure a good constitution in their Infants* . . . (New York, 1809), 7–11.

20. Watkins, *Maternal Solicitude*, 9–10; An American Matron, *The Maternal Physician, A Treatise on the Nurture and Management of Infants* . . . (New York, 1811), 8–9; William Buchan, *Advice to Mothers on the Subject of Their Own Health* . . . (Charleston, S.C., 1807), 31; Child, *The Mother's Book*, 4; Enos Hitchcock, *Memoirs of the Bloomsgrove Family. In a Series of Letters* . . . (Boston, 1790), 1 : 79–80. See also the discussion in Block, "American Feminine Ideals in Transition," 110–111.

21. Smith, *The Female Monitor*, 75; Lawrence Stone, *The Family, Sex and Marriage, in England 1500–1800* (New York, 1977), 427.

22. Cadogan, *An Essay Upon Nursing*, 33–34.

23. Ibid., p. 13; Watkins, *Maternal Solicitude*, 12–15.

24. Watkins, *Maternal Solicitude*, 12, 20–21; see also: Baker, *Cautions to Pregnant and Lying-in Women*, 11; Cadogan, *An Essay Upon Nursing*, 13–15; Rendle-Short, "Infant Management," 105–108.

25. Alcott, *The Young Mother*, 48–51; Barwell, *Infant Treatment*, 133–137; Kuhn, *The Mother's Role in Childhood Education*, 141–143; Sunley, "Early Nineteenth Century American Literature on Childrearing," 155. Quotation from Barwell.

26. Mary S. Gove, *Lectures to Ladies on Anatomy and Physiology* (Boston, 1842), 25–26, 263–264, 270.

27. Catharine Beecher, *A Treatise on Domestic Economy* (1841; reprint New York, 1977), 208; Gove, *Lectures to Ladies*, 289; Mrs. C. A. Hopkinson, *Hints for the Nursery, or The Young Mother's Guide* (Boston, 1863), 8, 17; Sigourney, *Letters to Mothers*, 73.

28. Sigourney, *Letters to Mothers*, 10.

29. Kathryn Kish Sklar, *Catharine Beecher: A Study in American Domesticity* (New York, 1973), 170–182; Thomas Woody, *Women's Education in the United States* (New York, 1929) 1 : 96–104, 460–465.

30. Kuhn, *The Mother's Role in Childhood Education*, 98–103.

31. Almira Phelps, "Observations Upon an Infant, During Its First Year. By a Mother," appended to Albertine Necker, *Progressive Education Commencing with the Infant*, trans. with notes and appendix by Emma Willard and Almira Phelps (Boston, 1835), 342.

32. Child, *The Mother's Book*, 10–11.

33. "Infant Education, According to the Principles of Pestalozzi," *Mother's Magazine* 4 (January 1836): 8–10; William Mavor, *The Mother's Catechism; or First Principles of Knowledge and Instruction for Very Young Children* (Leicester, Mass., 1815), Preface, 1–54 (entire book lists subjects to be taught, e.g., letters, numbers, money, weights, measures, time, planets and stars, and the weather).

34. Anonymous, *The Mother's Friend: or Directions for Forming the Mental and Moral Habits of Young Children* (New York, 1834), 135–136; Mavor, *Mother's Catechism*, 48.

35. Jacob Abbott, *The Little Philosopher, or The Infant School at Home* (Boston, 1833) cited in Kuhn, *The Mother's Role in Childhood Education*, 103–104.

36. Phelps, "Observations Upon an Infant," in Necker, *Progressive Education*, 342.

37. Ibid, 325.

38. Kuhn, *The Mother's Role in Childhood Education*, 74, and Chapter 4, "Religious and Moral Guide," (71–97). See also Block, "American Feminine Ideals in Transition," 112–113.

39. Joseph Lathrop, *Importance of Female Influence in the Support of Religion. A Sermon Delivered to a Charitable Female Association in West Springfield, May 15, 1810* (Springfield, Mass., 1810), 6. See also Jesse Appleton, *A Discourse delivered before the Members of the Portsmouth Female Asylum*, (Portsmouth, N.H., 1806), 6–10.

40. Abbott, *The Mother at Home*, 108.

41. Block, "American Feminine Ideals in Trasition," 113–114 on catechisms; "B. H. H.," "The Mother's Privilege," *Mother's Magazine* 1 (November 1833): 175–176; "Early Religious Impressions the Appropriate Business of Mothers," *Mother's Magazine* 111 (November 1835): 164–167. Quotation from "The Mother's Privilege."

42. George Burnap, *The Sphere and Duties of Woman*, 5th ed. (Baltimore, 1855), 111–112; "Early Religious Impressions the Appropriate Business of Mothers," 166.

43. Kuhn, *The Mother's Role in Childhood Education*, 80–83.

44. "B.," "The Great Helper," *Mother's Magazine* 1 (April 1833) : 61–62; Coxe, *Claims of the Country* 2 : 61, (see chapter entitled "Hints on the Moral Nurture of Youth").

45. "Habit of Prayer Early Formed," *Mother's Magazine* 1 (November 1833) : 176–177.

46. William Lyman, *A Virtuous Woman the Bond of Domestic Union, and the Source of Domestic Happiness. A Sermon Delivered at Lyme, Jan. 6, 1802* . . . (New London, Conn., 1802), 22.

47. William M. Thayer, "The Era for Mothers. A Prize Article," *Mother's Assistant* 21 (1851) : 129–146, especially 134–137.

48. "The Worth of Money," *Ladies' Magazine and Literary Gazette* 111 (February 1830) : 49–55.

49. *The American Lady's Preceptor: A Compilation of Observations, Essays and Poetical Effusions* . . . (Baltimore, 1813), 83 (Cornelia); Eliza Barton Lyman, *The Coming Woman: or The Royal Road to Physical Perfection. A Series of Medical Lectures* (Lansing, Mich., 1880), 268, 270; Reginald Newton, *Womanhood, Lectures on Woman's Work in the World* (New York, 1881), 149 (Augustine): Susan Tracy Rice, comp., *Mother's Day: Its History, Origin, Celebration, Spirit and Significance* . . . (New York, 1915), 227–290, section on "Mothers of the Famous" (Lincoln, Stevens, Emerson).

50. Abbott, *The Mother at Home*, 11 (Byron); Lyman, *The Coming Woman*, 269 (Byron); Sigourney, *Letters to Mothers*, 39–40 (Arnold). The Byron quotation is from Abbott.

51. Abbott, *The Mother at Home*, 10–11.

52. "The Integrity of Washington," *Mother's Magazine* 6 (August 1838), 184–188.

53. William M. Thayer, "The Mother of Washington," in Rice, comp., *Mother's Day*, 265–267; for a count of the appearances this story made in schoolbooks see Ruth Miller Elson, *Guardians of Tradition: American Schoolbooks in the Nineteenth Century* (Lincoln, Neb., 1964), 203, 307; also in Thayer, "Era for Mothers," 142–143.

54. Margaret C. Conkling, *Memoirs of the Mother and Wife of Washington*, rev. ed. (Auburn and Buffalo, N.Y., 1854), 57–59, quotation from p. 59; Marion Harland (Mary Terhune), *The Story of Mary Washington* (Boston, 1893), 124–128.

55. Harland, *The Story of Mary Washington*, 128.

56. Doris Faber, *The Mothers of American Presidents* (New York, 1968), 162–175. The

comparatively recent publication of this book suggests a hardy interest in presidential mothers.

57. D. Wise, "Praying Mothers," *Mother's Assistant* 9 (October 1846) : 81–82.

58. Abbott, *The Mother at Home*, 16; Sigourney, *Letters to Mothers*, 48–54. Quotation from Abbott.

59. Newton, *Womanhood*, 144; Elizabeth Torrey, *The Ideal of Womanhood, or Words to the Women of America* (Boston, 1858), 18–19. Quotation from Torrey.

60 "A Mother's Influence," *Mother's Magazine* 14 (1846) : 324.

61. John Todd, "Address to Mothers," *Mother's Magazine* 7 (November 1839): 247–249.

62. Herbert G. Gutman, "Work, Culture, and Society in Industrializing America, 1815–1919," *American Historical Review*, (June 1973) : 531–588. The continuous influx of immigrants with nonindustrialized work values in the nineteenth century meant the American work force was continually modernizing (i.e., learning the discipline of time, as opposed to task-created work) throughout the century. Gutman also discusses their enduring family ties.

63. Carl Bridenbaugh, *Cities in Revolt: Urban Life in America, 1743–1776* (1955; reprint New York, 1971); see Chapter 7, "Merchants and Craftsmen at Bay," 250–291, especially 281, 286–289; Chapter 4, "City People," 134–171; and Chapter 8, "Civic Improvements," 292–331. The classic description of late colonial entreprenurial activity and civic improvement exists in Benjamin Franklin, *The Autobiography of Benjamin Franklin*, ed. Henry Steele Commager (New York, 1944). See, on city improvements: library, pp. 79, 116–118; watch, fire company, battery building, pp. 127, 132–133; paving, pp. 141–142; street cleaning, pp. 143–145.

64. Victor S. Clark, *History of Manufactures in the United States* (New York, 1929), 1 : 319, 534–536; Samuel Rezneck, "The Rise and Early Development of Industrial Consciousness in the United States," *Journal of Economic and Business History*, 4 (August 1932) : 784–811; Alexander Hamilton, "Report on Manufactures," in *The Works of Alexander Hamilton*, ed. John C. Hamilton, v. 3 (New York, 1850), 192–204.

65. Richard D. Brown, "The Emergence of Urban Society in Rural Massachusetts, 1760–1820," *Journal of American History* 61 (June 1974) : 29–51, especially 47–48. See also Richard D. Brown, "Modernization and the Modern Personality in Early America, 1600–1865: A Sketch of a Synthesis," *Journal of Interdisiplinary History* 2 (1971–1972) : 201–208.

66. Simeon J. Crowther, "Urban Growth in the Mid-Atlantic States, 1785–1850," *Journal of Economic History* 36 (September 1976) : 627–631; Jeffery Williamson, "Urbanization in the American Northeast, 1820–1870," in *The Reinterpretation of American History*, ed. Robert Fogel and Stanley Engerman (New York, 1971), 428–429.

67. Clark, *History of Manufactures in the United States* 1 : 411. Clark points out that, with the exception of some Philadelphia factories, most manufactures did not utilize steam engines until after the 1850s, choosing to rely on waterpower instead: a significant reason why early factories were spread out along rivers outside the major cities. Crowther, "Urban Growth in the Mid-Atlantic States," 633, 643; Williamson, "Urbanization in American Northeast," 435–436.

68. Kenneth T. Jackson, "The Crabgrass Frontier: 150 Years of Suburban Growth in America," in *The Urban Experience*, ed. Raymond A. Mohl and James F. Richardson (Belmont, Calif., 1973), 206–207; Kenneth T. Jackson, "Urban Deconcentration in the Nineteenth Century: A Statistical Inquiry," in *New Urban History*, ed. Leo F. Schnore

(Princeton, N.J., 1975), 110–142; U.S. Department of the Interior, Bureau of the Census, "Population of Cities Having 25,000 Inhabitants or More in 1900, at Each Census: 1790–1900," *Twelfth Census of the United States, Taken in the Year 1900, Population, Part I* (Washington, D.C., 1901), 430–433. Population of New York City in 1860 after annexation: 814,000.

69. Douglas C. North, *The Economic Growth of the United States, 1790–1860* (1961; reprint New York, 1966), 5 : 159–163; George Rogers Taylor, *The Transportation Revolution, 1815–1860* (1951; reprint New York, 1968), chaps. 1–11, pp. 15–249, 396–398. As North explains, the census of 1860 ranked cotton goods as the nation's largest industry in terms of value of product. The cotton industry employed 114,955 people, but the boot and shoe industry, which was ranked third in the census, employed 123,026 people.

70. Theodore Parker, "A Sermon on the Public Function of Women, Preached at the Music-Hall, Boston, March 27, 1853," in *Commensurate With Her Capabilities and Obligations Are Woman's Rights. A Series of Tracts, Compromising Sixteen Articles, Essays, Addresses, and Letters of the Prominent Advocates of Woman's Larger Sphere of Action* (Syracuse, N.Y., 1853), 5.

71. Taylor, *The Transportation Revolution*, 211–214; Rolla Milton Tryon, *Household Manufactures in the United States, 1640–1860* (Chicago, 1917), 291–293, 304–305. Tryon is the most exhaustive history of household manufactures.

72. Tryon, *Household Manufactures*, 370–376. The system never assumed importance in Louisiana, Florida, Texas, Iowa, California, Minnesota, Oregon, and Kansas; settled between 1840 and 1860.

73. Hannah Hickok Smith's Account Book, 1821–1824, discussed in Cott, *The Bonds of Womanhood*, 43–44.

74. Edith Abbott, *Women in Industry: A Study in American Economic History* (New York, 1910), 90, 102, 124; Taylor, *The Transportation Revolution*, 216–220. Women's work in the two major nineteenth-century industries, textiles and shoes, is perceptively analyzed in Thomas Dublin, *Women at Work: The Transformation of Work and Community in Lowell, Massachusetts, 1820–1860* (New York, 1979), and Alan Dawley, *Class and Community: The Industrial Revolution in Lynn* (Cambridge, Mass., 1976).

75. Anna A. Rogers, *Why American Marriages Fail, and Other Papers* (Boston, 1909), 23–26. For an analysis of the development of women's role as shopper in the nineteenth century see Gunther Barth, *City People: The Rise of Modern City Culture in Nineteenth Century America* (New York, 1980), 110–147, Chapter 4; Cott, *Bonds of Womanhood*, 45.

76. Ruth Schwartz Cowan, *More Work for Mother: The Ironies of Household Technology from the Open Hearth to the Microwave* (New York, 1983), 40–68. Joann Vanek, "Time Spent in Housework," *Scientific American* 231 (November 1974): 116–120, compares statistics from 1925 to 1965, finding that the time devoted to housework remained stable. See also Beecher, *A Treatise on Domestic Economy*, especially chapters on "Cleanliness," "Washing," "Whitening, Cleansing, and Dying," "On the Care of Parlors," "On the Care of Kitchens," "On the Care of Chambers and Bedrooms," and "How to Wash Dishes."

77. Mary Lee to Hannah Lowell, May 25, 1811, and Mary Lee to Henry Lee, Sept. 1, 1813, in Frances Rollins Morse, ed., *Henry and Mary Lee: Letters and Journals* (Boston, 1926), 103, 152. Cott, *Bonds of Womanhood*, 46–51, discusses Lee and other women and analyzes relationships between greater population density and commercial development (1780–1835), greater reliance on purchasing power, and more attention to child-rearing.

78. Kenneth Jackson, "Urban Deconcentration in the Nineteenth Century: A Statistical Inquiry," in Schnore, ed., *The New Urban History*, 125–140.

79. Abbott, *The Mother at Home*, 155–157; Burnap, *Sphere and Duties of Woman*, 111; Coxe, *Claims of the Country 3 : 5–6;* "Infant Education," *The American Ladies' Magazine* 11 (February 1829): 89–90; summary of didactic literature in Jeffrey, "Family History," 164–167. Quotations from "Infant Education."

80. Mrs. Samuel McCune Lindsay, "The Suburban Child," *The Pedagogical Seminary* 16 (1909): 499–500, was among the first to write of suburban children, who rarely saw their fathers during the day, as a social problem. She thought the suburb was abnormal during the day because it was "a manless community."

81. Abbott, *The Mother at Home*, 157–158; see also Mrs. Ann Taylor, *Practical Hints to Young Females on the Duties of a Wife, a Mother, and a Mistress of a Family.* (Boston, 1816 [from the Third London Edition] 154–155; "A Father's Influence in the Domestic Circle," *Mother's Magazine* 111 (August 1835) : 116–119; "The Father's Position and Influence," *Mother's Magazine* 21 (1853) : 346–347.

82. Jill Conway, "Perspectives on the History of Women's Education in the United States," *History of Education Quarterly* 14 (Spring 1974) : 4–12; Roberta Wein, "Women's Colleges and Domesticity, 1875–1918," *History of Education Quarterly* 14 (Spring 1974) : 31–47.

83. Mary Benson, *Women in Eighteenth Century America*, (New York, 1935) 11–133, (especially 33), 314–315.

84. Thomas Osborne, *An Enquiry into the Duties of the Female Sex* (Philadelphia, 1798), 14–16, 35–44, 156; Benson, *Women in Eighteenth Century America*, 94–95.

85. Alice Lee Shippen to Anne Shippen Livingston, September 22, 1777, in Ethel Armes, ed., *Nancy Shippen, Her Journal Book, The International Romance of a Young Lady of Fashion of Colonial Philadelphia with Letters to Her and About Her* (Philadelphia, 1935), 41; Stone, *The Family, Sex and Marriage*, 343–360.

86. Ann D. Gordon, "The Young Ladies Academy of Philadelphia," in Berkin and Norton, *Women of America*, 84–86; Marion Lansing, *Mary Lyon Through Her Letters* (Boston, 1937), 15–37; Harriet Webster Marr, *The Old New England Academies, Founded Before 1826* (New York, 1959), 1–18, 97–106; Woody, *Women's Education* 1 : 329–459.

87. Mary Beth Norton has quantified information from *Notable American Women: A Biographical Dictionary* (Cambridge, Mass., 1971) on biographies from before 1810, which shows the "dramatic shift" in educational opportunity for women in the early Republic. An average of 65 percent of biographies of women born between 1770 and 1809 had advanced education. See Norton, *Liberty's Daughters* (Boston, 1980) 287–289.

88. Maris A. Vinovskis and Richard M. Bernard, "Beyond Catharine Beecher: Female Education in the Antebellum Period," *Signs* 4 (Summer 1978) : 856–866.

89. Vinovskis and Bernard, "Beyond Catharine Beecher," 867; Lockridge, *Literacy in Colonial New England*, 38–43; Arthur M. Schlesinger, Jr., *The Rise of the City, 1878–1898* (1933; reprint Chicago, 1961), 171–172.

90. Norton, *Liberty's Daughters*, 262–263.

91. Benson, *Women in Eighteenth Century America*, 314–315; Norton, *Liberty's Daughters*, 270–272.

92. Benjamin Rush, "Thoughts Upon Female Education, Accomadated to the Present State of Society, Manners, and Government, in the United States of America, July 28, 1787," in *Essays, Literary, Moral and Philosophical*, 2d ed. (Philadelphia, 1806), 75–92; see Benson, *Women in Eighteenth Century America*, 137, 143, for evaluation of Rush's influence.

93. Linda K. Kerber, "Daughters of Columbia: Educating Women for the Republic, 1787–1805," in *The Hofstadter Aegis, a Memorial* (New York, 1974), 36–59, ed. Stanley Elkins and Eric McKitrick; Linda K. Kerber, "The Republican Mother: Women and the Enlightenment—An American Perspective," *American Quarterly* 28 (Summer 1976) : 187–204.

94. Catharine Beecher, *Suggestions Respecting Improvements in Education, Presented to the Trustees of the Hartford Female Seminary, and Published at Their Request* (Hartford, Conn., 1829), 53–54.

94. Mrs. A. J. Graves, *Woman in America, Being an Examination Into the Moral and Intellectual Condition of American Female Society* (New York, 1841), 183–184, 195–196.

96. Daniel Webster, "Influence of Woman, from a Speech at Richmond," in *The Prose Writers of America . . .*, ed. Rufus Wilmot Griswold, rev. ed. (Philadelphia, 1870), 185.

97. William Alcott, *The Young Wife, or Duties of Woman in the Marriage Relation* (Boston, 1837), 306–308; Beecher, *Suggestions Respecting Improvements in Education*, 7; Catharine Beecher, *Woman Suffrage and Woman's Profession* (Hartford, Conn., 1871), 25–26; Emma Willard, *A Plan for Improving Female Education. A Reprint of the Second Edition of 1819* (Middlebury, Vt., 1918), 19, 20.

98. *A Sermon to Young Women: Republished from the Virginia Evangelical and Literary Magazine* (Richmond, Va., 1819); Graves, *Woman in America*, 66–68; Mrs. Townshend Stith, *Thoughts on Female Education* (Philadelphia, 1831), 16–18; Willard, *A Plan for Improving Female Education*, 6.

CONCLUSION

1. Eugene Becklard, M.D., *Physiological Mysteries and Revelations in Love . . .* (New York, 1842), 37.

2. Wilson H. Grabhill, Clyde V. Kiser, and Pascal K. Whelpton, "A Long View," in *The American Family in Social-Historical Perspective*, ed. Michael Gordon (New York, 1973); J. Potter, "The Growth of Population in America, 1700–1860," in *Population in History, Essays in Historical Demography*, ed. David V. Glass and David E. C. Eversley (Chicago, 1965); Robert Wells, "Demographic Change and the Life Cycle of American Families," in *The Family in History, Interdisciplinary Essays*, ed. Theodore K. Rabb and Robert I. Rotberg (New York, 1971).

3. Janet Farrell Brodie, "Contraception in Victorian America: The Dissemination of Semi-Licit Knowledge," paper presented at the Berkshire Conference of Women Historians, June 1976; Wilson Yates, "Birth Control Literature and the Medical Profession in Nineteenth Century America," *Journal of the History of Medicine and the Allied Sciences* 31 (January 1976) : 42–54.

4. Norman E. Himes, *Medical History of Contraception* (Baltimore, 1936), 224.

5. Charles Knowlton, M.D., *Fruits of Philosophy, or the Private Companion of Adult People*, 4th ed. (Philadelphia, 1839), 81–82.

6. Ibid., 88.

7. Ibid., 31.

8. F. Harrison Doane, *The Young Married Lady's Private Medical Guide*, 4th ed. (Boston, 1854), 231.

9. Henry C. Wright, *The Unwelcome Child; or The Crime of Undesigned Maternity* (Boston, 1860). See also Wesley Grindle, M.D., *New Medical Revelations, Being a Popular Work on the Reproductive System, Its Debility and Diseases* (Philadelphia, 1857), 167.

10. Wright, *Unwelcome Child*, 85–87.

11. James Reed, *From Private Vice to Public Virtue: The Birth Control Movement and American Society Since 1830* (New York, 1978), 10.

12. Ibid., 37–39.

13. John C. King, "Ethics and Methods of Preventing Conception," *Southern California Practitioner* 14 (1899) : 272–278.

14. Walter Channing, *A Treatise on Etherization in Childbirth. Illustrated by Five Hundred and Eighty-one Cases* (Boston, 1848).

15. For a good summary of the early use of anesthetics see Richard W. and Dorothy C. Wertz, *Lying-In: A History of Childbirth in America* (New York, 1977), 117–118.

16. Ibid., 150–154.

17. Haven Emerson and Anna C. Phillips, *Hospitals and Health Agencies of San Francisco, 1923* (San Francisco, 1923), 5.

18. *Harper's Weekly*, February 15, 1902, cited in James Harrar, *The Story of the Lying-in Hospital of New York* (New York, 1938), 52.

19. "Report of the Attending Physician," *Annual Report of the New England Hospital for Women and Children, 1865* (Boston, 1865), 13.

20. *Annual Report of the Society of the Lying-in Hospital of New York, 1901* (New York, 1901), 14.

21. Opinion of Justice David J. Brown, *Muller* v. *Oregon* (1908), reprinted in Richard Hofstadter, *Great Issues in American History* (New York, 1958), 2 : 270.

22. U.S. Department of Labor, Children's Bureau, *Save the Youngest, Seven Charts on Maternal and Infant Mortality, with Explanatory Comment*, Publication No. 61 (1918), 3.

23. *Society of the Lying-in Hospital of New York, Annual Report, 1921* (New York, 1921), 19.

24. Alice Weld Tallant, MS, "Maternal Mortality," in Alice Weld Tallant manuscript collection, Sophia Smith Collection, Smith College.

25. James Reed, *From Private Vice to Public Virtue: The Birth Control Movement in American Society Since 1830* (New York, 1978), 123–128.

26. Ellsworth Huntington and Leon F. Whitney, *The Builders of America* (New York, 1927), 303.

27. Dorothy Canfield Fisher, *Mothers and Children* (New York, 1914), 252.

Index